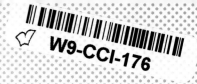

EVOLVE REACH ADMISSION ASSESSMENT EXAM REVIEW

Second edition

HESI

Contributing Authors

Louise Ables, MS
Phil Dickison, PhD(C), RN
Jean Flick, MS, RN
Mary Hinds, PhD, RN
Judy Hyland, MS, RN
Susan Morrison, PhD, RN
Bernice Rohlich, MS
John Tollett, BS
Deborah L. Walker, MS
Sherry Lutz Zivley, PhD

Editors

Donna Boyd
Elizabeth Saccoman, BA

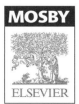

MOSBY
ELSEVIER

EVOLVE REACH ADMISSION ASSESSMENT EXAM REVIEW

Second edition

HESI

Contributing Authors
Louise Ables, MS
Phil Dickison, PhD(C), RN
Jean Flick, MS, RN
Mary Hinds, PhD, RN
Judy Hyland, MS, RN
Susan Morrison, PhD, RN
Bernice Rohlich, MS
Anne Tollett, BS
John Tollett, BS
Deborah L. Walker, MS
Sherry Lutz Zivley, PhD

Editors
Donna Boyd
Elizabeth Saccoman, BA

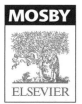
MOSBY
ELSEVIER

11830 Westline Industrial Drive
St. Louis, Missouri 63146

EVOLVE REACH ADMISSION ASSESSMENT EXAM REVIEW ISBN: 978-1-4160-5635-5
Second Edition
Copyright © 2009 by Mosby, Inc., an affiliate of Elsevier Inc.

Notice

Library of Congress Control Number: 2008920204

ISBN: 978-1-4160-5635-5

Managing Editor: Billi Sharp
Senior Developmental Editor: Mindy Hutchinson
Publishing Services Manager: Patricia Tannian
Project Manager: Jonathan M. Taylor
Design Direction: Mark Oberkrom

Printed in the United States of America

Last digit is the print number: 9 8 7 6 5 4

PREFACE

Congratulations on purchasing the *Evolve Reach Admission Assessment Exam Review* by HESI. This study guide was developed based on the Evolve Reach Admission Assessment Exam and is designed to assist students in preparation for entrance into higher education in a variety of health-related professions. Test items on the Evolve Reach Admission Assessment Exam are not specifically derived from this study guide. However, the content contained in the study guide provides an overview of the subjects tested on the Admission Assessment Exam and is meant to guide students' preparation for the exam. The *Evolve Reach Admission Assessment Exam Review* is written at the high school and beginning college levels and offers the basic knowledge that is necessary to be successful on the Admission Assessment Exam.

The Evolve Reach Admission Assessment consists of 10 different exams—eight academically oriented exams and two personally oriented exams. The academically oriented subjects consist of

- Mathematics
- Reading
- Vocabulary
- Grammar
- Biology
- Chemistry
- Anatomy and Physiology
- Physics

The chapters include conversion tables and practice problems in the Mathematics chapter; step-by-step explanations in the Reading and Grammar chapters; a substantial list of words used in health professions in the Vocabulary chapter; rationales and sample questions in the Biology, Chemistry, and Physics chapters; and helpful terminology in the Anatomy and Physiology chapter. Also included throughout the exam review are "HESI Hint" boxes, which are designed to offer students a suggestion, an example, or a reminder pertaining to a specific topic.

The personally oriented exams consist of a Learning Style assessment and a Personality Profile. These exams are intended to offer students insights about their study habits, learning preferences, and dispositions relating to academic achievement. Students generally like to take these exams for the purpose of personal insight and discussion. Because they take only approximately 15 minutes each to complete, the school may include these exams in their administration of the Admission Assessment Exam.

Schools can choose to administer any one or all of these exams provided by the Admission Assessment. For example, programs that do not require biology, chemistry, anatomy and physiology, or physics for entry into the program would not administer those Admission Assessment science-oriented exams.

The Evolve Reach Admission Assessment Exam has been used by colleges, universities, and health-related institutions as part of the selection and placement process for applicants and newly admitted students for approximately ten years.

Study Hints

It is always a good idea to prepare for any exam. When you begin to study for the *Admission Assessment Exam*, make sure you allocate adequate time and do not feel rushed. Set up a schedule that provides an hour or two each day to review material in the *Evolve Reach Admission Assessment Exam Review*. Mark the time you set aside on a calendar to remind yourself when to begin to study each day. Review the material for each section in the *Evolve Reach Admission Assessment Exam Review* that is relevant to your particular field of the healthcare professions. Complete the practice questions at the end of each chapter. If you are having trouble with the practice questions for a particular section, then review that content in the study guide again. It may also be helpful to go back to your textbook and class notes for additional review.

Test-Taking Hints

1. Read each question carefully and completely. Make sure you understand what the question is asking.

2. Identify the key words or phrases in the question. These words or phrases will provide critical information about how to answer the question.
3. Rephrase the question in your words.
   a. Ask yourself, "What is the question really asking?"
   b. Eliminate nonessential information from the question.
   c. Sometimes writers use terminology that may be unfamiliar to you. Do not be confused by a new writing style.
4. Rule out options (if they are presented).
   a. Read all of the responses completely.
   b. Rule out any options that are clearly incorrect.
   c. Mentally mark through incorrect options in your head.
   d. Differentiate between the remaining options, considering your knowledge of the subject.
5. Computer tests do not allow an option for skipping questions and returning to them later. Practice answering every question as it appears.

Do not second-guess yourself. TRUST YOUR ANSWERS.

CONTENTS

MATHEMATICS

M embers of the health professions use math every day to calculate medication dosages, radiation limits, nutritional needs, mental status, intravenous drip rates, intake and output, and a host of other requirements related to their clients. Safe and effective care is the goal of all who work in the health professions. Therefore it is essential that students entering the health professions be able to understand and make calculations using whole numbers, fractions, decimals, and percentages.

The purpose of this chapter is to review the addition, subtraction, multiplication, and division of whole numbers, fractions, decimals, and percentages. Mastery of these basic mathematic functions is an integral step toward a career in the health professions.

Basic Addition and Subtraction

Vocabulary

Digit: A numeral (e.g., the number 7 is a digit).

Place Value: Each digit in a number occupies a position; that position is called its place value.

(Modified from Macklin D, Chernecky CC, Infortuna H: *Math for clinical practice*, St Louis, 2005, Mosby.)

> **HESI Hint**
> I ten = 10 ones
> I hundred = 100 ones
> I thousand = 1000 ones

BASIC ADDITION

Example

462 + 133

$$\begin{array}{r} 462 \\ + 133 \\ \hline 595 \end{array}$$

Steps

1. Line up the digits according to place value.
2. Add the digits starting from right to left:
   - Ones: 2 + 3 = 5
   - Tens: 6 + 3 = 9
   - Hundreds: 4 + 1 = 5

ADDITION WITH REGROUPING

Example

835 + 559

$$\begin{array}{r} {}^{1} \\ 835 \\ + 559 \\ \hline 1{,}394 \end{array}$$

Steps

1. Line up the digits according to place value.
2. Add:

- Ones: $5 + 9 = 14$
  - Carry the 1 to the tens place, which is one place to the left.
- Tens: $1 + 3 + 5 = 9$
- Hundreds: $8 + 5 = 13$

BASIC SUBTRACTION

Example

$5,234 - 4,112$

$$\begin{array}{r} 5,234 \\ -\ 4,112 \\ \hline 1,122 \end{array}$$

Steps

1. Line up the digits according to place value.
2. Subtract:
   - Ones: $4 - 2 = 2$
   - Tens: $3 - 1 = 2$
   - Hundreds: $2 - 1 = 1$
   - Thousands: $5 - 4 = 1$

SUBTRACTION WITH REGROUPING

Example

$457 - 29$

$$\begin{array}{r} \overset{4\ 17}{4\cancel{5}\cancel{7}} \\ -\ 2\,9 \\ \hline 4\,2\,8 \end{array}$$

Steps

1. Align the digits according to place value.
2. Subtract:
   - Ones: $7 - 9$
     - Must borrow 1 from the 5 in the tens place: $17 - 9 = 8$
   - Tens: $4 - 2 = 2$
   - Hundreds: $4 - 0 = 4$

Sample Problems

Add or subtract in each of the following problems as indicated.
1. $1,803 + 156 =$
2. $835 + 145 =$
3. $1,372 + 139 =$
4. $123 + 54 + 23 =$
5. $673 - 241 =$
6. $547 - 88 =$
7. $222 - 114 =$
8. $12,478 - 467 =$

9. Jeff walks 5 miles west then turns north and walks 8 miles. How far has Jeff walked?
10. Julie picks 26 tomatoes from the tomato plants in her garden. She gives seven tomatoes to her next-door neighbor. How many tomatoes does Julie have now?

Basic Multiplication (Whole Numbers)

Vocabulary

Product: The answer to a multiplication problem.

> **HESI Hint** • Remember, the placeholders help keep the problem aligned. If you do not skip a space, the answer will be incorrect. Below is an example of a well-aligned problem.
>
> $$
> \begin{array}{r}
> 24571 \\
> \times\,1233 \\
> \hline
> 73713 \rightarrow \text{Ones} \\
> 737130 \rightarrow \text{Tens} \\
> 4914200 \rightarrow \text{Hundreds} \\
> +24571000 \rightarrow \text{Thousands} \\
> \hline
> 30{,}296{,}043
> \end{array}
> $$

Examples

Example 1

23×5

$$
\begin{array}{r}
^{1} \\
23 \\
\times\ 5 \\
\hline
115
\end{array}
$$

Steps

1. Multiply one digit at a time.
2. Multiply 5×23.
   - Ones: $5 \times 3 = 15$
     Carry the 1 to the tens place, and write the 5 in the ones place.
   - Tens: $5 \times 2 = 10 + 1 = 11$

Example 2

623×45

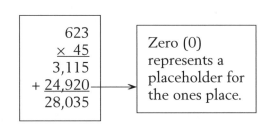

$$
\begin{array}{r}
623 \\
\times\ 45 \\
\hline
3{,}115 \\
+\ 24{,}920 \\
\hline
28{,}035
\end{array}
$$

Zero (0) represents a placeholder for the ones place.

Steps

1. Multiply 623×5.
   - $5 \times 3 = 15$
   - $5 \times 2 = 10 + 1$ (carried over) $= 11$
   - $5 \times 6 = 30 + 1$ (carried over) $= 31$ (does not need to be carried)
2. Multiply 623×4 (remember to line up the ones digit with the 4 by using zero as a placeholder).
   - $4 \times 3 = 12$
   - $4 \times 2 = 8 + 1 = 9$
   - $4 \times 6 = 24$
3. Add the two products together.
   - $115 + 24{,}920 = 28{,}035$ (the final product)

Example 3

301×451

```
      301
   × 451
      301
   15,050
+ 120,400
  135,751
```

Steps

1. Multiply 301×1.
   - $1 \times 1 = 1$
   - $1 \times 0 = 0$
   - $1 \times 3 = 3$
2. Multiply 301×5.
   - $5 \times 1 = 5$ (remember to use a zero for a placeholder)
   - $5 \times 0 = 0$
   - $5 \times 3 = 15$
3. Multiply 301×4.
   - $4 \times 1 = 4$
   - $4 \times 0 = 0$
   - $4 \times 3 = 12$
4. Add the three products together.
   - $301 + 15{,}050 + 120{,}400 = 135{,}751$ (the final product)

Sample Problem

Multiply in each of the following problems as indicated.
1. $846 \times 7 =$
2. $325 \times 6 =$
3. $653 \times 12 =$
4. $806 \times 55 =$
5. $795 \times 14 =$
6. $999 \times 22 =$
7. $582 \times 325 =$
8. $9438 \times 165 =$
9. Jan is preparing an examination for 29 students. Each student will have 30 questions, with no student having duplicate questions. How many questions will Jan need to prepare?

10. John is ordering lunch for the volunteers at the hospital. There are 12 units in the hospital, with 15 volunteers in each unit. How many lunches will John need to order?

Basic Division (Whole Numbers)

Vocabulary

Quotient: The answer to a division problem.
Dividend: The number being divided.
Divisor: The number by which the dividend is divided.

HESI Hint

$$5 \overline{)45} \quad \overset{9}{}$$

The 5 represents the **divisor**, the 45 represents the **dividend**, and the 9 represents the **quotient**. It is best not to leave a division problem with a remainder, but to end it as a fraction or decimal instead. To make the problem into a decimal, add a decimal point and zeros at the end of the dividend and continue. If a remainder continues to occur, round to the hundredths place.

Example:

$$233.547 \rightarrow 233.55 \text{ (the 7 rounds the 4 to a 5)}$$

Examples

Example 1

$40 \div 8$

$$8 \overline{)40} \quad \overset{5}{} \\ \underline{-40} \\ 0$$

Steps

1. Set up the problem (review the vocabulary section).
2. Use a series of multiplication and subtraction problems to solve a division problem.
3. $8 \times ? = 40$
   - Multiply: $8 \times 5 = 40$
   - Subtract: $40 - 40 = 0$
   - The quotient (or answer) is 5.

Example 2

$672 \div 6$

```
      112
   6)672
   -6↓↓
     07↓
    -6↓
     12
    -12
      0
```

Steps

1. Set up the problem.
2. Begin with the hundreds place.
    * $6 \times ? = 6$. We know $6 \times 1 = 6$; therefore place the 1 (quotient) above the 6 in the hundreds place (dividend). Place the other 6 under the hundreds place and subtract: $6 - 6 = 0$.
    *   Bring down the next number, which is 7; $6 \times ? = 7$. There is no number that can be multiplied by 6 that will equal 7 exactly, so try to get as close as possible without going over 7. Use $6 \times 1 = 6$ and set it up just like the last subtraction problem: $7 - 6 = 1$.
    *   Bring down the 2 from the dividend, which results in the number 12 (the 1 came from the remainder of $7 - 6 = 1$).
    * $6 \times ? = 12$; $? = 2$. The two becomes the next number in the quotient. $12 - 12 = 0$. There is not a remainder.
    *   The quotient (or answer) is 112.

Example 3

$174 \div 5$

```
      34.8
   5)174.0
   -15↓↓
     24↓
   - 20↓
      40
   - 40
      0
```

Steps

1. Set up the problem.
2. 5 does not divide into 1 but does divide into 17.
3. $5 \times 3 = 15$. Write the 3 in the quotient. (It is written above the 7 in 17 because that is the last digit in the number.)
    * $5 \times 3 = 15$
    * $17 - 15 = 2$
4. Bring the 4 down. Combine the 2 (remainder from $17 - 15$) and 4 to create 24.

5. Five does not divide evenly into 24; therefore try to get close without going over.
   - $5 \times 4 = 20$
   - $24 - 20 = 4$
6. There is a remainder of 4, but there is not a number left in the dividend. Add a decimal point and zeros and continue to divide.
7. The quotient (or answer) is 34.8 (thirty-four and eight tenths).

Sample Problems

Divide in each of the following problems as indicated.
1. $132 \div 11 =$
2. $9,618 \div 3 =$
3. $2,466 \div 2 =$
4. $325 \div 13 =$
5. $5,024 \div 8 =$
6. $3,705 \div 5 =$
7. $859 \div 4 =$
8. $6,987 \div 7 =$
9. There are 350 pieces of candy in a large jar. Ben wants to give the 25 campers in his group an even amount of candy. How many pieces of candy will each camper receive?
10. Edie has 132 tulip bulbs. She wants to plant all of the tulip bulbs in 12 rows. How many tulip bulbs will Edie plant in each row?

Addition and Subtraction of Decimals

Vocabulary

Place Value: Regarding decimals, numbers to the right of the decimal point have different terms from the whole numbers to the left of the decimal point. Each digit in a number occupies a position; that position is called its *place value*.

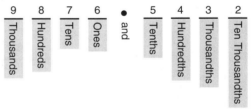

(Modified from Macklin D, Chernecky CC, Infortuna H: *Math for clinical practice*, St Louis, 2005, Mosby.)

HESI Hint • The word *and* stands for the decimal when writing a number in words.
Example: 5.7 (five and seven tenths)

Examples

Example 1

$2.6 + 3.1$

$$\begin{array}{r} 2.6 \\ + 3.1 \\ \hline 5.7 \end{array}$$

Steps

1. Align the decimal points.
2. Add the tenths together: $6 + 1 = 7$
3. Add the ones together: $3 + 2 = 5$
4. Final answer: 5.7 (five and seven tenths)

Example 2

5 + 12.34

```
  12.34
+  5.00
  17.34
```

Steps

1. Align the decimal points.
   - It might be difficult to align the 5 because it does not have a decimal point. Remember that after the ones place, there is a decimal point. To help with organization, add zeros (placeholders). Example: 5 = 5.00
2. Add the hundredths: $4 + 0 = 4$
3. Add the tenths: $3 + 0 = 3$
4. Add the ones: $2 + 5 = 7$
5. Add the tens: $1 + 0 = 1$
6. Final answer: 17.34 (seventeen and thirty-four hundredths).

Example 3

7.21 − 4.01

```
  7.21
− 4.01
  3.20
```

Steps

1. Align the decimal points
2. Subtract the hundredths: $1 − 1 = 0$
3. Subtract the tenths: $2 − 0 = 2$
4. Subtract the ones: $7 − 4 = 3$
5. Final answer: 3.20 (three and twenty hundredths)

Example 4

12 − 8.99

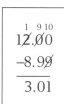

Steps

1. Align the decimal points.
2. Because 12 is a whole number, add a decimal point and zeros.
3. 0.00 − 0.99 cannot be subtracted; therefore 1 must be borrowed from the 12 and regrouped.

4. The ones become 1, the tenths become 9, and the hundredths become 10.
5. Subtract the hundredths: $10 - 9 = 1$
6. Subtract the tenths: $9 - 9 = 0$
7. Subtract the ones: $11 - 8 = 3$
   - 1 was borrowed from the tens in order to subtract the 8.
8. Final answer: 3.01 (three and one hundredth)

Sample Problems

Solve each of the following decimal problems as indicated.
1. $9.2 + 7.55 =$
2. $2.258 + 64.58 =$
3. $892.2 + 56 =$
4. $22 + 3.26 =$
5. $8.5 + 7.55 + 14 =$
6. $18 - 7.55 =$
7. $31.84 - 2.430 =$
8. $21.36 - 8.79 =$
9. Bill has 2.5 vacation days left for the rest of the year and 1.25 sick days left. If Bill uses all of his sick days and his vacation days, how many days will he have off work?
10. Erin has 6.25 peach pies. She gives Rose 3.75 of the peach pies. How many pies does Erin have left?

Multiplication of Decimals

Vocabulary

Place Value: Regarding decimals, numbers to the right of the decimal point have different terms from the whole numbers to the left of the decimal point. Each digit in a number occupies a position; that position is called its *place value*.

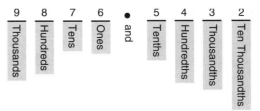

(Modified from Macklin D, Chernecky CC, Infortuna H: *Math for clinical practice*, St Louis, 2005, Mosby.)

Examples

Example 1

75.7×2.1

$$
\begin{array}{r}
75.7 \\
\times\ 2.1 \\
\hline
757 \\
+\ 15140 \\
\hline
158.97
\end{array}
$$

1 decimal place
+ 1 decimal place
---
2 decimal places

Move the decimal two places to the left in the final product.

Steps

1. Multiply 757×21 (do not worry about the decimal until the final product has been calculated).
2. Starting from the right, count the decimal places in both numbers and add together (two decimal places).
3. Move to the left two places, and then place the decimal.

Example 2

0.002×3.4

0.002	3 decimal places
× 3.4	+ 1 decimal place
0008	4 decimal places
+ 00060	
0.0068	Move four places to the left.

Steps

1. Multiply 2×34.
2. Starting from the right, count the decimal places in both numbers and add together (four decimal places).
3. Move to the left four places, and then place the decimal.

Example 3

3.41×7

3.41	2 decimal places
× 7	+ 0 decimal places
23.87	2 decimal places
	Move two places to the left.

Steps

1. Multiply 341×7.
2. Starting from the right, count the decimal places in both numbers and add together (two decimal places).
3. Move to the left two places, and then place the decimal.

Sample Problems

Multiply the decimals in the following problems as indicated.

1. $0.003 \times 4.23 =$
2. $98.26 \times 8 =$
3. $8.03 \times 2.1 =$
4. $250.1 \times 25 =$
5. $0.1364 \times 2.11 =$
6. $8.23 \times 4 =$
7. $0.058 \times 64.2 =$
8. $794.23 \times .001 =$
9. Jenny lost 3.2 lb each month for 6 months. How much weight has Jenny lost?
10. Richard wants to make 2.5 recipes of sugar cookies. Each recipe calls for 1.75 cups of sugar. How many cups of sugar will Richard need for 2.5 batches of cookies?

Division of Decimals

Vocabulary

Quotient: The answer to a division problem.
Dividend: The number being divided.
Divisor: The number by which the dividend is divided.

$$5\overline{)45} = 9$$

5 is the divisor, 45 is the dividend, and 9 is the quotient.
Place Value: Regarding decimals, numbers to the right of the decimal point have different terms than whole numbers.

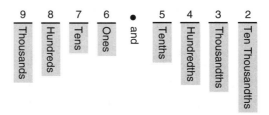

9	8	7	6	•	5	4	3	2
Thousands	Hundreds	Tens	Ones	and	Tenths	Hundredths	Thousandths	Ten Thousandths

(Modified from Macklin D, Chernecky CC, Infortuna H: *Math for clinical practice*, St. Louis, 2005, Mosby.)

> **HESI Hint •** The number 25 is a whole number. Though this number could be written 25.0, decimals are usually not displayed after a whole number.

Examples

Example 1

34 ÷ 2.5

$$\begin{array}{r} 13.6 \\ 2.5\overline{)34.0_{,}0} \\ -25\downarrow\downarrow \\ \overline{90}\downarrow \\ -75\downarrow \\ \overline{150} \\ -150 \\ \overline{0} \end{array}$$

Steps

1. Set up the division problem.
2. Move the decimal point in 2.5 one place to the right, making it a whole number.
3. What is done to one side must be done to the other side. Move the decimal point one place to the right in 34, making it 340, and then bring the decimal point up into the quotient.
4. Divide normally.
   - 25 × 1 = 25
   - Subtract: 34 − 25 = 9

- Bring down the zero to make 90.
- $25 \times 3 = 75$. This is as close to 90 as possible without going over.
- Subtract: $90 - 75 = 15$
- Add a zero to the dividend and bring it down to the 15, making it 150.
- $25 \times 6 = 150$
- $150 - 150 = 0$

5. The quotient is 13.6.

Example 2

$2.468 \div 0.2$

```
      12.34
0.2)2.4.68
  -2↓↓↓
   04↓↓
  - 4↓↓
    06↓
   -6↓
    08
   -8
    0
```

Steps

1. Set up the division problem.
2. Move the decimal point in 0.2 over one place to the right, making it a whole number. 0.2 is now 2.
3. Move the same number of spaces in the dividend. 2.468 is now 24.68.
4. Bring the decimal point up to the quotient in the new position.
5. Divide normally.

Example 3

$0.894 \div 0.05$

```
        17.88
0.05)0.89.40
   -5↓ ↓↓
    39↓↓
   - 35↓↓
     44↓
   - 40↓
      40
    -40
      0
```

Steps

1. Set up the division problem.
2. Move the decimal point in the divisor until it is a whole number. 0.05 is now 5.

3. Move the decimal in the dividend the same number of spaces as was moved in the divisor. 0.894 is now 89.4
4. Divide normally.

Sample Problems

Divide the decimals in the following problems as indicated.
1. $48 \div 0.4 =$
2. $144 \div 0.6 =$
3. $3.75 \div 0.4 =$
4. $56.2 \div 0.2 =$
5. $2.6336 \div 0.32 =$
6. $591 \div 0.3 =$
7. $0.72 \div 0.8 =$
8. $0.132 \div 0.11 =$
9. Stewart has 56 acres of land. He wants to divide the land into plots of 0.25 acres. How many plots of land will Stewart have after he divides the 56 acres?
10. Donna has 4.2 liters of fertilizer. If each pecan tree needs 0.7 liters of fertilizer and Donna uses all of the fertilizer, how many pecan trees does Donna have?

Fractions

This section discusses vocabulary, improper fractions, reducing, least common denominators (LCDs), and mixed numbers.

Vocabulary

$$\frac{\text{Numerator (part)}}{\text{Denominator (whole)}}\text{Fraction bar}$$

Numerator: The top number in a fraction.
Denominator: The bottom number in a fraction.
Common Denominator: Two or more fractions having the same denominator.
Least Common Denominator: The smallest multiple that two numbers share.

Example

1. $\frac{21}{7}$ is solved using division: $7\overline{)21}^{\,3}$
2. The top number goes inside the box. The bottom number goes outside the box.
3. The answer is 3.

Description

- The numerator is the top number of the fraction. It represents the part or pieces.
- The denominator is the bottom number of the fraction. It represents the total or whole amount.
- The fraction bar is the line that separates the numerator and the denominator.

An improper fraction occurs when the numerator is larger than the denominator. An improper fraction should always be reduced or made into a mixed number.

REDUCING FRACTIONS USING THE GREATEST COMMON FACTOR

Description

Factor: A number that divides evenly into another number.

Example

Factors of 12:

- $1 \times 12 = 12$
- $2 \times 6 = 12$
- $3 \times 4 = 12$

12 {1, 2, 3, 4, 6, 12}: Listing the factors helps determine the greatest common factor between two or more numbers.

$$\frac{1}{2} = \frac{2}{4}, \frac{3}{6}, \frac{4}{8}, \frac{5}{10}, \frac{6}{12}, \frac{7}{14}, \frac{8}{16}, \frac{9}{18}, \frac{10}{20}$$

All represent a half.

Reducing fractions can also be called reducing a fraction to its lowest terms or simplest form.

$$1 = \frac{1}{1}, \frac{2}{2}, \frac{3}{3}, \frac{4}{4}, \frac{5}{5}, \frac{6}{6}, \frac{7}{7}, \frac{8}{8}, \frac{9}{9}, \frac{10}{10}$$

Reduce $\frac{7}{21}$

Factors of 7 and 21:

7 {1, 7}

21 {1, 3, 7, 21}

The greatest common factor is 7; therefore divide the numerator and denominator by 7.

$$\frac{7}{21} \div \frac{7}{7} = \frac{1}{3}$$

Reduce $\frac{12}{20}$

Factors of 12 and 20:

12 {1, 2, 3, 4, 6, 12}

20 {1, 2, 4, 5, 10, 20}

The greatest common factor is 4 (they do have 1 and 2 in common, but the greatest factor is needed).

$$\frac{12}{20} \div \frac{4}{4} = \frac{3}{5}$$

LEAST COMMON DENOMINATOR

The LCD is the smallest multiple that two numbers share. Determining the LCD is an essential step in the addition, subtraction, and ordering of fractions.

Examples

Example 1

Find the LCD for $\frac{3}{4}$ and $\frac{7}{9}$.

Steps

1. List the multiples (multiplication tables) of each denominator.
   - 4: $4 \times 1 = 4$, $4 \times 2 = 8$, $4 \times 3 = 12$, $4 \times 4 = 16$, $4 \times 5 = 20$, $4 \times 6 = 24$, $4 \times 7 = 28$, $4 \times 8 = 32$, $4 \times 9 = 36$, $4 \times 10 = 40$
   - 4 {4, 8, 12, 16, 20, 24, 28, 32, 36, 40}—this will be the standard form throughout for listing multiples.
   - 9 {9, 18, 27, 36, 45, 54, 63, 72, 81, 90}
2. Compare each for the least common multiple.
   - 4 {4, 8, 12, 16, 20, 24, 28, 32, 36, 40}
   - 9 {9, 18, 27, 36, 45, 54, 63, 72, 81, 90}
3. The LCD between 4 and 9 is 36 ($4 \times 9 = 36$ and $9 \times 4 = 36$).

Example 2

Find the LCD for $\frac{3}{12}$ and $\frac{1}{8}$.

Steps

1. List the multiples of each denominator, and find the common multiples.
   - 12 {12, 24, 36, 48, 60, 72, 84, 96, 108, 120}
   - 8 {8, 16, 24, 32, 40, 48, 56, 64, 72, 80}
   - Find the **least** (or smallest) common multiple.
2. The LCD between 12 and 8 is 24 ($12 \times 2 = 24$ and $8 \times 3 = 24$).

CHANGING IMPROPER FRACTIONS INTO MIXED NUMBERS

An improper fraction has a larger numerator than denominator.

Example

$$\frac{17}{5} \rightarrow 5\overline{)17} \rightarrow 3\frac{2}{5}$$
$$\phantom{\frac{17}{5} \rightarrow 5)} \frac{15}{2}$$

Steps

1. Fractions cannot be left in this form; therefore turn it into a mixed number through division. (The top number [numerator] goes in the box; the bottom number [denominator] stays out.)
2. The 3 becomes the whole number.
3. The remainder becomes the numerator.
4. The denominator stays the same.

CHANGING MIXED NUMBERS INTO IMPROPER FRACTIONS

A mixed number has a whole number and fraction combined.

Example

$$5\frac{2}{3} \rightarrow 5\frac{+2}{\times 3} = (5 \times 3) + 2 = 17 \rightarrow \frac{17}{3}$$

Steps

1. To make a mixed number into an improper fraction, multiply the denominator and whole number together, then add the numerator.
2. Place this new numerator over the denominator, which stays the same in the mixed number.

ADDITION OF FRACTIONS

Addition with Common Denominators

Example

$$\frac{3}{7} + \frac{2}{7} = \frac{5}{7}$$

Steps

1. Add the numerators together: $3 + 2 = 5$.
2. The denominator stays the same, 7.
3. Answer: $\frac{5}{7}$ (five sevenths).

Addition with Unlike Denominators

Example

$$\frac{1}{5} + \frac{7}{10}$$

$$\frac{1 \times 2}{5 \times 2} = \frac{2}{10}$$

$$\frac{7 \times 1}{10 \times 1} = \frac{7}{10}$$

$$\frac{2}{10} + \frac{7}{10} = \frac{9}{10}$$

Steps

1. Find the LCD by listing the multiple of each denominator.
   - 5 (5, 10, 15, 20, 25, 30)
   - 10 (10, 20, 30, 40, 50)
   - The LCD is 10.
2. If the denominator is changed, the numerator must also be changed by the same number. Do this by multiplying the numerator and denominator by the same number.

$$\frac{1 \times 2}{5 \times 2} = \frac{2}{10}$$

3. Because the denominator of the second fraction is 10, no change is necessary.
4. Add the numerators together, and keep the common denominator.
5. Reduce the fraction if necessary.

Addition of Mixed Numbers

Example

$$1\frac{1}{4} + 2\frac{8}{10}$$

$$1\frac{1 \times 5}{4 \times 5} = 1\frac{5}{20}$$

$$2\frac{8 \times 2}{10 \times 2} = 2\frac{16}{20}$$

$$1\frac{5}{20} + 2\frac{16}{20} = 3\frac{21}{20} = 4\frac{1}{20}$$

Steps

1. Find a common denominator of 4 and 10 by listing the multiples of each.
   - 4 (4, 8, 12, 16, 20)
   - 10 (10, 20, 30)
2. Calculate the new numerator of each fraction to correspond to the changed denominator.
3. Add the whole numbers together, and then add the numerators together. Keep the common denominator 20.
4. The numerator is larger than the denominator (improper); change the answer to a mixed number (review vocabulary if necessary).

Sample Problems

Add the fractions in the following problems as indicated.

1. $\dfrac{1}{12} + \dfrac{5}{12} =$

2. $\dfrac{7}{21} + \dfrac{10}{21} =$

3. $\dfrac{1}{2}+\dfrac{4}{5}=$

4. $\dfrac{5}{7}+\dfrac{3}{14}=$

5. $\dfrac{4}{5}+\dfrac{6}{7}=$

6. $7\dfrac{1}{8}+2\dfrac{4}{12}=$

7. $5\dfrac{2}{9}+1\dfrac{2}{9}=$

8. $12\dfrac{1}{21}+3\dfrac{1}{3}=$

9. Mary is going to make a birthday cake. She will need 1⅔ cups of sugar for the cake and 2½ cups of sugar for the frosting. How many cups of sugar will Mary need for the frosted birthday cake?

10. Greg is installing crown molding on two sides of a room. The length of one wall is 11¾ feet. The length of the other wall is 13⅞ feet. How much crown molding will Greg install in the room?

SUBTRACTION OF FRACTIONS

Vocabulary

Numerator: The top number in a fraction.
Denominator: The bottom number in a fraction.
Common Denominator: Two or more fractions having the same denominator.
Least Common Denominator: The smallest multiple that two numbers share.
Factor: A number that divides evenly into another number.

Example
$12 \div 6 = 2$ (6 and 2 are factors of 12).

HESI Hint • Fractions as a whole:

$\dfrac{15}{15} = 1$ (one whole)

Notice in the example under "Borrowing from Whole Numbers" that we added 15 to both the numerator and the denominator. We did this because it is one whole and it is the same denominator.

SUBTRACTING FRACTIONS WITH COMMON DENOMINATORS

Example

$$\dfrac{7}{9}-\dfrac{4}{9}=\dfrac{3}{9}=\dfrac{1}{3}$$

Steps

1. Subtract the numerators: $(7 - 4 = 3)$.
2. Keep the same denominator.
3. Reduce the fraction by dividing by the greatest common factor:

$$\frac{3}{9} \div \frac{3}{3} = \frac{1}{3}$$

SUBTRACTING FRACTIONS WITH UNLIKE DENOMINATORS

Example

$$\frac{5}{12} - \frac{1}{8} = ?$$

$$\frac{5 \times 2}{12 \times 2} = \frac{10}{24}$$

$$\frac{1 \times 3}{8 \times 3} = \frac{3}{24}$$

$$\frac{10}{24} - \frac{3}{24} = \frac{7}{24}$$

Steps

1. Find the LCD by listing the multiples of each denominator.
   - 12 {12, 24, 36, 48}
   - 8 {8, 16, 24, 32}
   - The LCD is 24.
2. Change the numerator to reflect the new denominator. (What is done to the bottom must be done to the top of a fraction.)
3. Subtract the new numerators: $10 - 3 = 7$. The denominator stays the same.

BORROWING FROM WHOLE NUMBERS

Example

$$5\frac{2}{3} - 3\frac{4}{5}$$

$$5\frac{2 \times 5}{3 \times 5} = 5\frac{10}{15}$$

$$^4\cancel{5}\frac{10}{15} + \frac{15}{15} = 4\frac{25}{15}$$

$$3\frac{4 \times 3}{5 \times 3} = 3\frac{12}{15}$$

$$4\frac{25}{15} - 3\frac{12}{15} = 1\frac{13}{15}$$

Steps

1. Find the LCD.
2. Twelve cannot be subtracted from 10; therefore 1 must be borrowed from the whole number, making it 4, and the borrowed 1 must be added to the fraction.

3. Add the original numerator to the borrowed numerator: $10 + 15 = 25$.
4. Now the whole number and the numerator can be subtracted.

Sample Problems

Subtract the fractions in the following problems as indicated.

1. $\dfrac{3}{20} - \dfrac{2}{20} =$

2. $\dfrac{28}{37} - \dfrac{17}{37} =$

3. $\dfrac{17}{25} - \dfrac{3}{5} =$

4. $\dfrac{31}{54} - \dfrac{5}{9} =$

5. $1\dfrac{9}{10} - \dfrac{1}{5} =$

6. $15\dfrac{7}{18} - \dfrac{3}{9} =$

7. $25\dfrac{1}{7} - 12\dfrac{5}{7} =$

8. $30\dfrac{1}{2} - 13\dfrac{3}{4} =$

9. Alan is making a table. The table will be 6 ½ feet long and 4 feet wide. The board for the table is 7⅞ feet long and 4 feet wide. How much of the board will Alan need to cut off?
10. McKenna has 1⅔ cups of milk. She gives Mark ¾ cup of milk to make a cake. How much milk will McKenna have left?

MULTIPLICATION OF FRACTIONS

Vocabulary

Numerator: The top number in a fraction.
Denominator: The bottom number in a fraction.
Factor: A number that divides evenly into another number.

> **HESI Hint •** "Multiplying fractions is no problem. Top times top and bottom times bottom."
> To change an improper fraction in a mixed number, divide the numerator by the denominator.
>
> $$\frac{20}{13} \rightarrow 13\overline{)20} \rightarrow 1\frac{7}{13}$$
> $$\phantom{\frac{20}{13} \rightarrow 13)}\underline{13}$$
> $$\phantom{\frac{20}{13} \rightarrow 13)}07$$
>
> The quotient becomes the whole number. The remainder becomes the numerator, and the denominator stays the same.

Examples

Example 1

$$\frac{4}{5} \times \frac{1}{2}$$

$$\frac{4}{5} \times \frac{1}{2} = \frac{4}{10} = \frac{2}{5}$$

Steps

1. Multiply the numerators together: $4 \times 1 = 4$.
2. Multiply the denominators together: $5 \times 2 = 10$.
3. Reduce the product by using the greatest common factor: $\frac{4}{10} \div \frac{2}{2} = \frac{2}{5}$.

Example 2

$$5 \times \frac{4}{13}$$

$$\frac{5}{1} \times \frac{4}{13} = \frac{20}{13} = 1\frac{7}{13}$$

Steps

1. Make the whole number 5 into a fraction by placing a 1 as the denominator.
2. Multiply the numerators: $5 \times 4 = 20$.
3. Multiply the denominators: $1 \times 13 = 13$.
4. Change the improper fraction into a mixed number.

Example 3

$$2\frac{1}{8} \times 7\frac{5}{6}$$

$$2\frac{1}{8} \times 7\frac{5}{6}$$

$$\frac{17}{8} \times \frac{47}{6} = \frac{799}{48}$$

$$\frac{799}{48} = 16\frac{31}{48}$$

Steps

1. Change the mixed numbers into improper fractions.

$$2\frac{+1}{\times 8} = (2 \times 8) + 1 = 17 \rightarrow \frac{17}{8}$$

$$7\frac{+5}{\times 6} = (7 \times 6) + 5 = 47 \rightarrow \frac{47}{6}$$

2. Multiply the numerators and denominators together.
   - $17 \times 47 = 799$ (numerator)
   - $8 \times 6 = 48$ (denominator)

- Change the improper fraction into a mixed number.

$$48\overline{)799} \begin{array}{r} 16 \\ \hline \end{array} = 16\frac{31}{48}$$

$$\begin{array}{r} 48 \\ \hline 319 \\ 288 \\ \hline 31 \end{array}$$

Sample Problems

Multiply the following fractions and reduce the product to the lowest common denominator.

1. $\dfrac{3}{5} \times \dfrac{2}{3} =$

2. $\dfrac{7}{9} \times \dfrac{1}{9} =$

3. $6 \times \dfrac{4}{5} =$

4. $1\dfrac{2}{5} \times 5 =$

5. $2\dfrac{1}{7} \times 1\dfrac{3}{4} =$

6. $4\dfrac{4}{5} \times 1\dfrac{4}{6} =$

7. $3\dfrac{1}{3} \times 2 =$

8. $1\dfrac{8}{12} \times 4\dfrac{1}{2} =$

9. Alec has six friends who each give him 2¾ pieces of gum. How many pieces of gum does Alec have now?

10. Rick rides 11⅛ miles in an hour with his bike in second gear going uphill. If Rick rides downhill in fourth gear he goes 2½ times faster. How many miles will Rick go in an hour downhill in fourth gear?

DIVISION OF FRACTIONS

Vocabulary

Numerator: The top number in a fraction.
Denominator: The bottom number in a fraction.
Reciprocals: Pairs of numbers that when multiplied together equal 1.
Factor: A number that divides evenly into another number.

HESI Hint • "Dividing fractions, don't ask why, inverse the second fraction and multiply."

Example:

$$\frac{1}{2} \div \frac{3}{8} \quad \text{Inverse} \quad \frac{3}{8} \rightarrow \frac{8}{3}$$

Then multiply $\dfrac{1}{2} \times \dfrac{8}{3}$

$$\frac{3}{8} \rightarrow \frac{8}{3} \quad \frac{3}{8} \times \frac{8}{3} = \frac{24}{24} = 1$$

These two numbers are reciprocals of each other, because when they are multiplied together, they equal 1.

Examples

Example 1

$$\frac{1}{2} \div \frac{3}{8}$$

$$\frac{1}{2} \div \frac{3}{8}$$

$$\frac{1}{2} \times \frac{8}{3} = \frac{8}{6}$$

Steps

1. Inverse (or take the reciprocal) of the second fraction: $\dfrac{3}{8} \rightarrow \dfrac{8}{3}$.
2. Rewrite the new problem and multiply.
   - $1 \times 8 = 8$ (numerator)
   - $2 \times 3 = 6$ (denominator)

Example 2

$$1\frac{5}{6} \div \frac{3}{4}$$

$$1\frac{5}{6} \div \frac{3}{4}$$

$$\frac{11}{6} \div \frac{3}{4}$$

$$\frac{11}{6} \times \frac{4}{3} = \frac{44}{18}$$

$$2\frac{8}{18} = 2\frac{4}{9}$$

Steps

1. Change the mixed number into an improper fraction: $1\dfrac{5}{6} = (1 \times 6) + 5 = \dfrac{11}{6}$.
2. Rewrite the new problem with the improper fraction.
3. Inverse the second fraction.

4. Multiply the numerators and the denominators together.
   - $11 \times 4 = 44$ (numerators)
   - $6 \times 3 = 18$ (denominators)
5. Change the improper fraction into a mixed number. Reduce the mixed number.

   Example 3

   $12 \div 2\dfrac{3}{8}$

   $$\dfrac{12}{1} \div \dfrac{19}{8}$$

   $$\dfrac{12}{1} \times \dfrac{8}{19} = \dfrac{96}{19}$$

   $$5\dfrac{1}{19}$$

Steps

1. Change the whole number into a fraction and the mixed number into an improper fraction.
2. Inverse the second fraction.
3. Multiply the numerators and then denominators together.
   - $12 \times 8 = 96$
   - $1 \times 19 = 19$
4. Change the improper fraction into a mixed number.

Sample Problems

Divide the fractions in the following problems and reduce to the lowest common denominator.

1. $\dfrac{4}{5} \div \dfrac{1}{7} =$

2. $\dfrac{12}{15} \div \dfrac{3}{5} =$

3. $\dfrac{7}{8} \div \dfrac{1}{6} =$

4. $1 \div \dfrac{1}{5} =$

5. $8 \div \dfrac{1}{4} =$

6. $2\dfrac{1}{4} \div \dfrac{1}{6} =$

7. $10 \div 3\dfrac{1}{3} =$

8. $12\dfrac{1}{3} \div 2 =$

9. Danny has 11¼ cups of chocolate syrup. He is going to make chocolate sundaes for his friends. Each sundae will have ¾ cup of chocolate. How many sundaes can Danny make?
10. Jenny has 8⅓ yards of ribbon. She is making bows for her bridesmaids. Each bow has ⅚ yard of ribbon. How many bridesmaids does Jenny have for her wedding?

CHANGING FRACTIONS TO DECIMALS

Vocabulary

Fraction Bar: The line between the numerator and denominator. The bar is another symbol for division.
Terminating Decimal: A decimal that is not continuous.

> **HESI Hint** • "Top goes in the box, the bottom goes out."
> This is a helpful saying in remembering that the numerator is the dividend and the denominator is the divisor.
>   If the decimal does not terminate, continue to the thousandths place and then round to the hundredths place.
> **Example:**
>
> $$7.8666 \rightarrow 7.87$$
>
>   If the number in the thousandths place is 5 or greater, round the number in the hundredths place to the next higher number.
>   However, if the number in the thousandths place is less than 5, do not round up the number in the hundredths place.

Examples

Example 1

Change $\dfrac{3}{4}$ to a decimal.

$$
\begin{array}{r}
0.75 \\
4\overline{)3.00} \\
-28\downarrow \\
\hline
20 \\
-20 \\
\hline
0
\end{array}
$$

Steps

1. Change the fraction into a division problem.
2. Add a decimal point after the 3 and add two zeros.
   • Remember to raise the decimal into the quotient area.
3. The answer is a terminating decimal; therefore adding additional zeros is not necessary.

Example 2

Change $\dfrac{5}{8}$ to a decimal.

```
    0.625
8)5.000
  -48↓↓
    20↓
   -16↓
     40
    -40
      0
```

Steps

1. Change the fraction into a division problem.
2. Add a decimal point after the 5 and add two zeros.
   • Remember to raise the decimal into the quotient area.
3. If there is still a remainder, add another zero to the dividend and bring it down.
4. The decimal terminates at the thousandths place.

Example 3

Change $\frac{2}{3}$ to a decimal.

```
    0.6666
3)2.0000
  -18↓↓↓
    2 0↓↓
   -18↓↓
     20↓
    -18↓
      20
```

Steps

1. Change the fraction into a division problem.
2. After the 2, add a decimal point and two zeros.
3. The decimal continues (does not terminate); therefore round to the hundredths place: $0.666 \rightarrow 0.67$.

It can also be written as $0.\overline{6}$ (the line is placed over the number that repeats).

Example 4

Change $2\frac{3}{5}$ to a decimal.

```
    0.60
5)3.00
  -30↓
    00
   -0
     0
```

Steps

1. Change the fraction into a division problem.

2. After the 3, add a decimal and two zeros.
3. Place the whole number in front of the decimal: 2.6.

Sample Problems

Change the following fractions into decimals and round it to the nearest thousandth.

1. $\dfrac{1}{5}$

2. $\dfrac{2}{5}$

3. $\dfrac{3}{8}$

4. $\dfrac{4}{5}$

5. $\dfrac{1}{3}$

6. $1\dfrac{1}{2}$

7. $\dfrac{3}{10}$

8. $2\dfrac{7}{8}$

9. $11\dfrac{11}{15}$

10. $\dfrac{12}{25}$

Changing Decimals to Fractions

Vocabulary

Place Value: Numbers to the right of the decimal point have different terms than do the whole numbers.

9	8	7	6	•	5	4	3	2
Thousands	Hundreds	Tens	Ones	and	Tenths	Hundredths	Thousandths	Ten Thousandths

(Modified from Macklin D, Chernecky CC, Infortuna H: *Math for clinical practice*, St Louis, 2005, Mosby.)

Examples

Example 1
Change 0.9 to a fraction.

$$0.9 \rightarrow \frac{9}{10}$$

Steps

Knowing place values makes it very simple to change decimals to fractions.
1. The last digit is located in the tenths place; therefore the 9 becomes the numerator.
2. 10 becomes the denominator.

Example 2
Change 0.02 to a fraction.

$$0.02 \rightarrow \frac{2}{100} = \frac{1}{50}$$

Steps

1. The 2 is located in the hundredths place.
2. The numerator becomes 2, and 100 becomes the denominator.
3. Reduce the fraction.

Example 3
Change 0.25 to a fraction.

$$0.25 \rightarrow \frac{25}{100} = \frac{1}{4}$$

Steps

1. Always look at the last digit in the decimal. In this example the 5 is located in the hundredths place.
2. The numerator becomes 25, and 100 becomes the denominator.
3. Reduce the fraction.

Example 4
Change 3.055 into a fraction.

$$3.055 \rightarrow 3\frac{55}{1000} \rightarrow 3\frac{11}{200}$$

Steps

1. The 5 is located in the thousandths place.
2. The numerator becomes 55 and 1,000 becomes the denominator. The 3 is still the whole number.
3. Reduce the fraction.

Sample Problems

Change the following decimals into fractions and reduce to the lowest common denominator.

1. 0.08 =
2. 0.025 =
3. 0.125 =
4. 0.17 =
5. 0.3 =
6. 2.75 =
7. 7.07 =
8. 12.0001 =
9. 3.48 =
10. 0.275 =

Ratios and Proportions

Vocabulary

Ratio: A relationship between two numbers.
Proportion: Two ratios that have equal values.

HESI Hint • Ratios can be written several ways.

As a fraction: $^5/_{12}$
Using a colon: 5:12
In words: 5 to 12

Proportions can be written two ways.

$$\frac{5}{12} = \frac{25}{60}$$

$$5:12 :: 25:60$$

NOTE: The numerator is listed first, then the denominator.

Examples

Example 1
Change the decimal to a ratio

$$0.025 \to \frac{25}{1000} \to \frac{1}{40} \to 1:40$$

Steps

1. Change the decimal to a fraction.
2. Reduce the fraction.
3. The numerator is the first listed number.
4. Then write the colon.
5. Finally, place the denominator after the colon.

Example 2
Change the fraction to a ratio.

$$\frac{5}{6} = 5:6$$

Steps

1. The numerator is the first listed number.
2. Then write the colon.
3. Finally, place the denominator after the colon.

Example 3

Solve the proportion (find the value of x).

$$7:10 :: 14:x$$

$$\frac{7}{10} = \frac{14}{x}$$

$$\frac{7}{10} \, \substack{\times 2 \\ \times 2} \, \frac{14}{x}$$

$$\frac{7}{10} = \frac{14}{x}$$

$$x = 20$$

Steps

1. Rewrite the proportion as a fraction. (this might help to see the solution).
2. Note that $7 \times 2 = 14$; therefore $10 \times 2 = 20$.
   - Multiply 14×10 (two diagonal numbers). The answer is 140.
   - $140 \div 7 = 20$ (Divide the remaining number.)
3. The answer is 20.

Example 4

Solve the proportion (find the value of x).

x:63 :: 24:72.

$$\frac{x}{63} = \frac{24}{72}$$

$$\frac{x}{63} = \frac{24}{72}$$

$$24 \times 63 = 1512$$
$$1{,}512 \div 72 = 21$$
$$x = 21$$

Steps

1. Rewrite the proportion as a fraction.
2. Multiply the diagonal numbers: $24 \times 63 = 1512$.
3. Divide the answer (1,512) by the remaining number: $1{,}512 \div 72 = 21$.
4. The value for x is 21.

Example 5

Solve the proportion.

240:60 :: x:12.

$$\frac{240}{60} = \frac{x}{12}$$

$$\frac{240}{60} = \frac{x}{12}$$

$$x = 48$$

Steps

1. Rewrite the proportion as a fraction.
2. Multiply the diagonal numbers together: $240 \times 12 = 2,880$.
3. Divide the answer (2,880) by the remaining number: $2,880 \div 60 = 48$.
4. The answer to x is 48.

Sample Problems

Change the following fractions to ratios:

1. $\frac{22}{91}$
2. $\frac{19}{40}$

Solve the following for x:

3. $7:5 :: 91:x$
4. $7:9 :: x:63$
5. $x:15 :: 120:225$
6. $15:x :: 3:8$
7. $360:60 :: 6:x$
8. $x:81 :: 9:27$
9. John buys 3 bags of chips for $4.50. How much will it cost John to buy five bags of chips?
10. The recipe states that 4 cups of sugar will make 144 cookies. How many cups of sugar are needed to make 90 cookies?

Percentages

VOCABULARY

Percent: Per hundred (part per hundred).

9	8	7	6	•	5	4	3	2
Thousands	Hundreds	Tens	Ones	and	Tenths	Hundredths	Thousandths	Ten Thousandths

(Modified from Macklin D, Chernecky CC, Infortuna H: *Math for clinical practice*, St Louis, 2005, Mosby.)

Examples

Example 1

Change the decimal to a percent: 0.13 → 13%.

Steps

1. Move the decimal point to the right of the hundredths place (two places).
2. Put the percent sign behind the new number.

Example 2

Change the decimal to a percent: 0.002 → 0.2%.

Steps

1. Move the decimal point to the right of the hundredths place (two places—always!).
2. Put the percent sign behind the new number. It is still a percent; it is just a very small percent.

Example 3

Change the percent to a decimal: 85.4% → 0.854.

Steps

1. Move the decimal two spaces away from the percent sign (to the left).
2. Drop the percent sign; it is no longer a percent, but a decimal.

Example 4

Change the percent to a decimal: 75% → 0.75.

Steps

1. The decimal point is not visible but is always located after the last number.
2. Move the decimal two spaces away from the percent sign (toward the left).
3. Drop the percent sign; the number is no longer a percent, but a decimal.

Example 5

Change the fraction to a percent: $\dfrac{5}{6}$

$$
\begin{array}{r}
.833 \\
6\overline{)5.000} \\
-4\,8\downarrow\downarrow \\
\hline
20\downarrow \\
-\quad18\downarrow \\
\hline
20
\end{array}
$$

0.833 → 83.3%

Steps

1. Change the fraction into a division problem and solve.
2. Move the decimal behind the hundredths place in the quotient.
3. Place a percent sign after the new number.

Sample Problems

Change the following decimals to percents.
1. 0.98 =
2. 0.0068 =
3. 0.09 =

Change the following percents to decimals.
4. 58% =
5. 76.3% =
6. 0.03% =

Change the following fractions to percents.

7. $\dfrac{9}{10}$ =

8. $\dfrac{4}{5}$ =

9. $\dfrac{1}{6}$ =

10. $\dfrac{3}{8}$ =

USING THE PERCENT FORMULA

HESI Hint • The word *of* usually indicates the **whole** portion of the percent formula.

Percent formula:

$$\frac{\text{Part}}{\text{Whole}} = \frac{\%}{100}$$

Using this formula will help in all percent problems in which there is an unknown (solving for *x*).

Examples

Example 1

What is 7 out of 8 expressed as a percent?

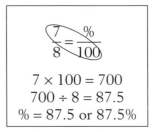

$$\frac{7}{8} = \frac{\%}{100}$$

7 × 100 = 700
700 ÷ 8 = 87.5
% = 87.5 or 87.5%

Steps

1. Rewrite the problem using the percent formula.
2. Multiply the diagonal numbers together: 7 × 100 = 700.
3. Divide by the remaining number: 700 ÷ 8 = 87.5%.

Example 2

What is 68% of 45?

$$\frac{x}{45} = \frac{68}{100}$$

$$45 \times 68 - 3,060$$
$$3,060 \div 100 = 30.6$$
$$x = 30.6$$

Steps

1. Rewrite the problem using the percent formula.
2. "Of 45:" 45 is the whole.
3. Multiply the diagonal numbers together: $68 \times 45 = 3,060$.
4. Divide by the remaining number: $3,060 \div 100 = 30.6$.
5. $x = 30.6$ (this is not a percent; it is the **part**).

Example 3

18 is 50% of what number?

$$\frac{18}{x} = \frac{50}{100}$$

$$18 \times 100 = 1800$$
$$1800 \div 50 = 36$$
$$x = 36$$

Steps

1. Rewrite the problem using the percent formula.
2. We are looking for the **whole** because *of* is indicating an unknown number.
3. Multiply the diagonal numbers together: $18 \times 100 = 1800$.
4. Divide by the remaining number: $1800 \div 50 = 36$.

Sample Problems

Solve the following percent problems.
1. What is 15 out of 75 as a percent?
2. What is 2 out of 50 as a percent?
3. What is 20 out of 100 as a percent?
4. What is 28% of 100?
5. What is 95% of 20?
6. What is 15.5% of 600?
7. The number 2 is 20% of what number?
8. The number 65 is 25% of what number?
9. The number 9 is 20% of what number?
10. The number 44 is 25% of what number?

Regular Time versus Military Time

Regular time uses the numbers 1 through 12 with the suffixes AM or PM to represent the hour in a 24-hour period. Military time uses the numbers 00 through 23 to represent the hour in a 24-hour period. The minutes and seconds in regular and military time are expressed the same way.

> **HESI Hint** • To convert to military time before noon, simply include a zero before the numbers 1 through 9 for AM. For example, 9:35 AM regular time converts to 0935 military time. The zero is not needed when converting 10 AM or 11 AM. If the time is after noon, simply add 12 to the hour number. For example, 1:30 PM regular time converts to 1330 military time (1 + 12 = 13). Midnight, or 12 AM, is converted to 0000. Noon, or 12 PM, is converted to 1200.

Table 1-1 summarizes the equivalents between military time and regular time. Military time is written with a colon between the minutes and seconds just as in regular time. It can also be expressed with a colon between the hours and the minutes.

Military time is written as follows:

hoursminutes:seconds   OR   **hours**:minutes:seconds

0932:24 hours   OR   09:23:24

1926:56 hours   OR   19:26:56 hours

Regular time is written as follows:

hours:minutes:seconds AM or PM

9:32:24 AM

7:26:56 PM

Sample Problems

Convert the following regular times to military times.
1. 12:00 AM =
2. 3:30 PM =
3. 11:19:46 AM =
4. 8:22:54 PM =
5. 4:27:33 PM =
6. 2:22:22 AM =

TABLE 1-1   Equivalents for Military Time and Regular Time

Military Time	Regular Time	Military Time	Regular Time
0000	12:00 AM (Midnight)	1200	12:00 PM (Noon)
0100	1:00 AM	1300	1:00 PM
0200	2:00 AM	1400	2:00 PM
0300	3:00 AM	1500	3:00 PM
0400	4:00 AM	1600	4:00 PM
0500	5:00 AM	1700	5:00 PM
0600	6:00 AM	1800	6:00 PM
0700	7:00 AM	1900	7:00 PM
0800	8:00 AM	2000	8:00 PM
0900	9:00 AM	2100	9:00 PM
1000	10:00 AM	2200	10:00 PM
1100	11:00 AM	2300	11:00 PM

Convert the following military times to regular times.
   7. 0603:45 hours
   8. 1200:00 hours
   9. 15:16:42 hours
  10. 16:18:00 hours
  11. 10:33:29 hours
  12. 21:11:34 hours

Helpful Information to Memorize and Understand

Fractions, Decimals, and Percents

Fraction	Decimal	Percent
$\frac{1}{2}$	0.50	50%
$\frac{1}{4}$	0.25	25%
$\frac{3}{4}$	0.75	75%
$\frac{1}{5}$	0.20	20%
$\frac{2}{5}$	0.40	40%
$\frac{3}{5}$	0.60	60%
$\frac{4}{5}$	0.80	80%
$\frac{1}{8}$	0.125	12.5%
$\frac{3}{8}$	0.375	37.5%
$\frac{5}{8}$	0.625	62.5%
$\frac{7}{8}$	0.875	87.5%
$\frac{1}{3}$	$0.33\overline{3}$	33.3%
$\frac{2}{3}$	$0.66\overline{6}$	66.6%

Roman Numerals

I = I	XX = 20	M = 1,000
II = 2	XXX = 30	$\overline{V}$ = 5,000
III = 3	XL = 40	$\overline{X}$ = 10,000
IV = 4	L = 50	$\overline{L}$ = 50,000
V = 5	LX = 60	$\overline{C}$ = 100,000
VI = 6	LXX = 70	$\overline{D}$ = 500,000
VII = 7	LXXX = 80	$\overline{M}$ = 1,000,000
VIII = 8	XC = 90	
IX = 9	C = 100	
X = 10	D = 500	
XI = II		
Example 　2003 = MMIII		

Measurement Conversions

TEMPERATURE	
0° Celsius = 32° Fahrenheit (the freezing point of water)	
100° Celsius = 212° Fahrenheit (the boiling point of water)	

LENGTH	
Metric	*English*
I kilometer = 1,000 meters	I mile = 1,760 yards
I meter = 100 centimeters	I mile = 5,280 feet = 1.609 km
I centimeter = 10 millimeters	I yard = 3 feet
	I foot = 12 inches

VOLUME AND CAPACITY	
Metric	*English*
1 dm³ = — I liter = 1,000 milliliters	I gallon = 4 quarts
I milliliter = I cubic centimeter = 1 cm³	I gallon = 128 ounces
	I quart = 2 pints
	I pint = 2 cups
	I cup = 8 ounces
	I ounce = 30 milliliters (cubic centimeters) (fl oz)

WEIGHT AND MASS	
Metric	*English*
I kilogram = 1,000 grams	I ton = 2,000 pounds = 907.03 kg
I gram = 1,000 milligrams	I pound = 16 ounces = 0.454 kg (lb)
	I ounce = 28.35 grams (oz)

Answers to Sample Problems

Basic Addition and Subtraction

1. 1,959
2. 980
3. 1,511
4. 200
5. 432
6. 459
7. 108
8. 12,011
9. 13 miles
10. 19

Basic Multiplication (Whole Numbers)

1. 5,922
2. 1,950
3. 7,836
4. 44,330
5. 11,130
6. 21,978
7. 189,150
8. 1,557,270
9. 870
10. 180

Basic Division (Whole Numbers)

1. 12
2. 3,206
3. 1,233
4. 25
5. 628
6. 741
7. 214.75
8. 998.14
9. 14
10. 11

Addition and Subtraction of Decimals

1. 16.75
2. 66.838
3. 948.2
4. 25.26

5. 30.05
6. 10.45
7. 29.41
8. 12.57
9. 3.75
10. 2.5

Multiplication of Decimals

1. 0.01269
2. 786.08
3. 16.863
4. 6252.5
5. 0.287804
6. 32.92
7. 3.7236
8. 0.79423
9. 19.2
10. 4.375

Division of Decimals

1. 120
2. 240
3. 9.375
4. 281
5. 8.23
6. 1,970
7. 0.9
8. 1.2
9. 224
10. 6

Addition of Fractions

1. $\dfrac{1}{2}$

2. $\dfrac{17}{21}$

3. $1\dfrac{3}{10}$

4. $\dfrac{13}{14}$

5. $1\dfrac{23}{35}$

6. $9\dfrac{11}{24}$

7. $6\dfrac{4}{9}$

8. $15\dfrac{8}{21}$

9. $4\dfrac{1}{6}$

10. $25\dfrac{5}{8}$

Subtraction of Fractions

1. $\dfrac{1}{20}$

2. $\dfrac{11}{37}$

3. $\dfrac{2}{25}$

4. $\dfrac{1}{54}$

5. $1\dfrac{7}{10}$

6. $15\dfrac{1}{18}$

7. $12\dfrac{3}{7}$

8. $16\dfrac{3}{4}$

9. $1\dfrac{3}{8}$ feet

10. $\dfrac{11}{12}$ cups

Multiplication of Fractions

1. $\dfrac{2}{5}$

2. $\dfrac{7}{81}$

3. $4\frac{4}{5}$

4. 7

5. $3\frac{3}{4}$

6. 8

7. $6\frac{2}{3}$

8. $7\frac{1}{2}$

9. $16\frac{1}{2}$

10. $27\frac{13}{16}$

Division of Fractions

1. $5\frac{3}{5}$

2. $1\frac{1}{3}$

3. $5\frac{1}{4}$

4. 5

5. 32

6. $13\frac{1}{2}$

7. 3

8. $6\frac{1}{6}$

9. 15

10. 10

Changing Fractions to Decimals

1. 0.2
2. 0.4
3. 0.375
4. 0.8
5. $0.\bar{3}$
6. 1.5

7. 0.3   0.3
8. 2.875
9. 11.7333
10. 0.48

Changing Decimals to Fractions

1. $\frac{2}{25}$
2. $\frac{1}{40}$
3. $\frac{1}{8}$
4. $\frac{17}{100}$
5. $\frac{3}{10}$
6. $2\frac{3}{4}$
7. $7\frac{7}{100}$
8. $12\frac{1}{10000}$
9. $3\frac{12}{25}$
10. $\frac{11}{40}$

Ratios and Proportions

1. 22:91
2. 19:40
3. $x = 65$
4. $x = 49$
5. $x = 8$
6. $x = 40$
7. $x = 1$
8. $x = 27$
9. $x = \$7.50$
10. $x = 2.5$

Percentages

1. 98%
2. 0.68%

3. 9%
4. 0.58
5. 0.763
6. ~~3~~ 0.0003
7. 90%
8. 80%
9. 16.667%
10. 37.5%

Using the Percent Formula

1. 20%
2. 4%
3. 20%
4. 28
5. 19
6. 93
7. 10
8. 260
9. 45
10. 176

Regular Time versus Military Time

1. 0000 hours OR 00:00 hours
2. 1530 hours OR 15:30 hours
3. 1119:46 hours OR 11:19:46 hours
4. 2022:54 hours OR 20:22:54 hours
5. 1627:33 hours OR 16:27:33 hours
6. 0222:22 hours OR 02:22:22 hours
7. 6:03:45 AM
8. 12:00 PM OR Noon
9. 3:16:42 PM
10. 4:18 PM
11. 10:33:29 AM
12. 9:11:34 PM

READING

2

Written communication is one of the primary ways of giving and receiving information about clients in the health care setting. The client record, whether it is on paper or in a computer, is the written documentation of what is known about a client—the client's health care history, the evaluation or assessment, the diagnosis, the treatment, the care, the progress, and, finally, the outcome. The ability to read and understand what has been written is necessary for any student who wants to enter a health care profession.

The purpose of this chapter is to review reading skills. The skills described in this chapter include the following:

1. Identifying the main idea (both stated and implied)
2. Identifying supporting details
3. Finding the meaning of words in context
4. Identifying a writer's purpose and tone
5. Distinguishing between fact and opinion
6. Making logical inferences
7. Summarizing

Identifying the Main Idea

Identifying the main idea is the key to understanding what has been read and what needs to be remembered. First, identify the topic of the passage or paragraph by asking the question, "What is it about?" Once that question has been answered, ask, "What point is the author making about the topic?" If the reader understands the author's message about the topic, then the main idea has been identified.

In longer passages the reader might find it helpful to count the number of paragraphs used to describe what is believed to be the main idea statement. If the majority of paragraphs include information about the main idea statement the reader has chosen, then the reader is probably correct. However, if the answer chosen by the reader is mentioned in only one paragraph, then the main idea chosen is probably a detail.

Another helpful hint in identifying main ideas is to read a paragraph and then stop and summarize that paragraph. This type of active reading helps the reader focus on the content and will lessen the need for rereading the entire passage several times.

Some students find visualizing as they read very helpful in remembering details and staying focused. They picture the information they are reading as if it were being projected on a big-screen TV. If you do not already do this, try it. Informal classroom experiments have proven that on comprehension tests students who visualize while reading easily outscore their counterparts who do not visualize.

> **HESI Hint** • Main ideas can be found in the beginning, in the middle, or at the end of a paragraph or passage. Always check the introduction and conclusion for the main idea.

Finally, not all main ideas are stated. Identify unstated or implied main ideas by looking specifically at the details, examples, causes, and reasons given.

Again, asking the questions stated earlier will help in this task:
- What is the passage about? (Topic)
- What point is the author making about the topic? (Main idea)

Some experts like to compare the main idea with an umbrella covering all or most of the details in a paragraph or passage. The chosen main idea can be tested for accuracy by asking whether the other details will fit under the umbrella. The idea of an umbrella also helps visualize how broad a statement the main idea can be.

Identifying Supporting Details

Writing is made up of main ideas and details. Few would enjoy reading only a writer's main ideas. The details provide the interest, the visual picture, and the examples that sustain a reader's interest.

Often students confuse the author's main idea with the examples or reasons the author gives to support the main idea. These details give the reader a description, background, or simply more information to support the writer's assertion or main idea. Without these details, the reader would not be able to evaluate whether the writer has made his or her case, nor would the reader find it as interesting. In addition to examples, facts and statistics may be used.

The reader's job is to distinguish between the details, which support the writer's main idea, and the main idea itself. Usually the reader can discover clues to help identify details because often an author uses transition words such as *one, next, another, first,* or *finally* to indicate that a detail is being provided.

Finding the Meaning of Words in Context

Even the most avid of readers will come across words with unknown meaning. Identifying the correct meaning of these words may be the key to identifying the author's main idea and to fully comprehending the author's meaning. The reader can, of course, stop and use a dictionary for these words. However, that is usually neither the most efficient nor the most practical way to approach these unknown words.

There are other options the reader can use to find the meanings of unknown words, and these involve using context clues. The phrase *context clues* refers to the information provided by the author in the words or sentences surrounding the unknown word or words.

Some of the easiest context clues to recognize are as follows:

1. Definition—The author puts the meaning of the word in parentheses or states the definition in the following sentence.
2. Synonym—The author gives the reader another word that is more familiar but means the same as the unknown word.
3. Antonym—The author gives a word that means the opposite of the unknown word.

> **HESI Hint** • The reader needs to watch for clue words such as *although, but*, and *instead*, which sometimes signal that an antonym is being used.

4. Restatement—The author restates the unknown word in a sentence using more familiar words.
5. Examples—The author gives examples that clearly help the reader understand the meaning of the unknown word.
6. Explanation—The author gives more information about the unknown word, which better explains the meaning of the word.
7. Word structure—Sometimes simply knowing the meanings of basic prefixes, suffixes, and root words can help the reader make an educated guess about an unknown word.

> **HESI Hint** • When being tested on finding the meaning of a word in the context of a passage, look carefully at the words and sentences surrounding the unknown word. The context clues are usually there for the reader to uncover. Once the correct meaning has been chosen, test that meaning in the passage. It should make sense, and the meaning should be supported by the other sentences in the passage or paragraph.

Identifying a Writer's Purpose and Tone

The purposes or reasons for reading or writing are similar for the readers and writers. Readers read to be entertained, and authors write to entertain. Readers choose to read for information, and writers write to inform. However, in the area of persuasion, readers can be fooled into believing they are reading something objective when in fact the author is trying to manipulate the readers' thinking. That is why it is important for readers to ask the following questions:

1. Who is the intended audience?
2. Why is this being written?

If the writer is trying to change the reader's thinking, encourage the reader to buy something, or convince the reader to vote for someone, the reader can assume the writer's goal is to persuade. More evidence can be found to determine the writer's purpose by identifying specific words used within the passage. Words that are biased, or words that have positive or negative connotations, will often help the reader determine the author's reason for writing. (*Connotation* refers to the emotions or feelings that the reader attaches to words.)

If the writer uses a number of words with negative or positive connotations, they are usually trying to manipulate the reader's thinking about a person, place, or thing. Looking at the writer's choice of words also helps the reader determine the tone of the passage. (An author's *tone* refers to the attitude or feelings the author has about the topic.)

For example, if the author is writing about the Dallas City Council's decision to build waterways on the Trinity River bottom to resemble the San Antonio Riverwalk and describes this decision as being "inspired" and "visionary," the reader knows the author has positive feelings about the decision. The tone of this article is positive because the words *inspired* and *visionary* are positive words. The reader might also be aware that the author may be trying to manipulate the reader's thinking.

On the other hand, if the writer describes the council's decision as being "wasteful" and "foolhardy," the reader knows the author has negative feelings about the council's decision. The reader can determine that the tone is unfavorable because of the words the writer chose. Typically, articles with obvious positive or negative tones and connotations will be found on the opinion or editorial page of the newspaper.

Articles or books written to inform should be less biased, and information should be presented in factual format and with sufficient supporting data to allow readers to form their own opinions on the event that occurred.

Distinguishing between Fact and Opinion

A critical reader must be an active reader. A critical reader must question and evaluate the writer's underlying assumptions. An assumption is a set of beliefs that the writer has about the subject. A critical reader must determine whether the writer's statements are facts or opinions and whether the supporting evidence and details are relevant and valid. A critical reader is expected to determine whether the author's argument is credible and logical.

To distinguish between fact and opinion, the reader must understand the common definitions of those words. A fact is considered something that can be proven (either right or wrong). For example, at the time Columbus sailed for the New World, it was considered a scientific fact that the world was flat. Columbus proved the scientists wrong.

An opinion is a statement that cannot be proven. For example, "I thought the movie *Titanic* was the best movie ever made," is a statement of opinion. It is subjective; it is the writer's personal opinion. On the other hand, the following is a statement of fact: "More people saw the movie *Titanic* in 1997 than any other movie." This statement is a fact because it can be proven to be correct.

Again, the reader must look closely at the writer's choice of words in determining fact or opinion. Word choices that include measurable data and colors are considered factual or concrete words. "Frank weighs 220 pounds" and "Mary's dress is red" are examples of concrete words being used in statements of fact.

If the writer uses evaluative or judgmental words *(good, better, best, worst)*, it is considered a statement of opinion. Abstract words *(love, hate, envy)* are also used in statements of opinion. These include ideas or concepts that cannot be measured. Statements that deal with probabilities or speculations about future events are also considered opinions.

Making Logical Inferences

In addition to determining fact and opinion, a critical reader is constantly required to make logical inferences. An inference is an educated guess or conclusion drawn by the reader based on the available facts and information. Although this may sound difficult and sometimes is, it is done all the time. A critical reader does not always know whether the inference is correct, but the inference is made based on the reader's own set of beliefs or assumptions.

Determining inferences is a skill often referred to as *reading between the lines*. It is a logical connection that is based on the situation, the facts provided, and the reader's knowledge and experience. The key to making logical inferences is to be sure the inferences are supportable by evidence or facts presented in the reading. This often requires reading the passage twice so that details can be identified. Inferences are not stated in the reading, but are derived from the information presented and influenced by the reader's knowledge and experience.

Summarizing

Identifying the best summary of a reading selection is a skill most students find frustrating. Yet this skill can be mastered easily when the following three rules are used:

1. The summary should include the main ideas from the beginning, middle, and end of the passage.
2. The summary must be presented in sequence; it cannot move from the beginning to the end and then back to the middle.
3. The summary must have accurate information. Sometimes a test summary will deliberately include false information. In that case, the critical reader will automatically throw that test option out.

This type of question will typically take the longest for the student to answer, because to answer it correctly the student must go through each summary choice and locate the related information or main idea in the passage itself. Double-checking the summary choices is one way of proving that the reader has the best summary, because if the summary choice presents information that is inaccurate or out of order, the reader will automatically eliminate those choices.

> **HESI Hint** • Remember, the summary should include the main ideas of the passage, possibly with some major supporting details. It should never repeat the same main idea. Finally, it is a shortened version of the passage that includes all the important information, eliminating the unnecessary and redundant.

Sample Reading Questions*

According to news reports, more senior citizens are accruing credit card debt than ever before. One reason given for the increase is that many seniors simply did not save enough money for retirement. Another reason given is the high cost of prescription drugs that are not covered by Medicare. Although the possibility of a prescription drug benefit being added to Medicare was a big issue in the last presidential campaign, it does not appear that any legislation will be enacted soon.

Meanwhile, some seniors are spending 50% to 60% of their incomes on prescription drugs. With utilities, mortgages, and groceries, it is easy to see why some seniors are forced to use their credit cards. According to SRI Consulting Business Intelligence in Princeton, New Jersey, a research and consulting firm, the average debt of households headed by someone over 65 rose from $8000 in 1992 to $23,000 in 2000. That is an increase of 188%.

Another reason given for seniors ending up in so much debt is the fact that they don't understand how credit cards work, and when they simply pay the minimum, most of the payment goes toward interest. Whatever the reason, many seniors today have to abandon formerly held conservative attitudes toward debt and join the millions of Americans who buy on credit.

Congress should enact Medicare legislation that helps make prescriptive drugs more affordable for seniors. It doesn't seem fair that those who have worked hard all their lives should have to worry about finding enough money to pay their bills in their so-called golden years. Write your congressional representatives and encourage them to enact the appropriate legislation.

1. What is the main idea of the passage?
   A. The high cost of prescription drugs is a difficult burden for seniors to bear.
   B. Credit card debt for seniors rose 188% from 1992 to 2000.
   C. Senior citizens today did not save enough money for their retirement years.
   D. There are several reasons why many senior citizens today are in credit card debt.
2. Which of the following is not listed as a detail in the passage?
   A. Seniors did not save enough for retirement.
   B. Many seniors spend money gambling.
   C. The cost of prescription drugs is a drain on seniors' income.
   D. Seniors do not always understand how credit cards work.
3. What is the meaning of the word *accruing* as used in the first paragraph?
   A. Something that increases or accumulates
   B. Something that attaches itself likes a parasite
   C. Something that annoys
   D. Something that describes emotion
4. What is the author's primary purpose in writing this essay?
   A. To inform
   B. To persuade
   C. To entertain
   D. To analyze
5. Identify the overall tone of the essay.
   A. Encouraging
   B. Optimistic
   C. Pessimistic
   D. Angry

*This section was written before Medicare Part D was enacted by the U. S. Congress

Continued

Sample Reading Questions—cont'd

6. Which of the following statements is an opinion?
   A. More seniors are accruing credit card debt than ever before.
   B. The high cost of prescription drugs has added to the credit card debt of seniors.
   C. Congress should enact Medicare legislation to make prescription drugs more affordable.
   D. Some seniors get into debt because they do not understand how credit cards work.
7. Which statement would not be inferred by the reader?
   A. Some seniors are having a difficult time paying their bills.
   B. Seniors should not allow their children to use their credit cards.
   C. Some seniors did not plan well for their retirement.
   D. Some seniors have to use credit cards to pay for their food and other basic necessities.
8. Choose the best summary of the passage.
   A. Prescription costs are keeping seniors in credit card debt. Many seniors were not financially prepared for retirement. Some seniors do not understand how credit cards work. There has been a huge increase in credit card debt for households headed by seniors.
   B. More seniors have credit card debt than ever before. Some seniors do not understand how credit cards work. The high cost of prescription drugs has caused many to use their credit cards for basic necessities. Something needs to be done to help seniors enjoy their retirement years.
   C. The average debt for households headed by seniors has decreased in the last decade. Many seniors hold conservative attitudes about debt, but they are being forced to abandon their ideas out of necessity. Congress could help seniors by enacting legislation that would reduce the cost of prescription drugs.
   D. More seniors hold credit card debt than ever before. Reasons for this include the lack of adequate financial planning for retirement, the high cost of prescription drugs, and the misunderstanding of how credit cards work. Congress needs to enact legislation to help today's seniors with the high cost of prescription drugs.

Answers to Sample Reading Questions

1. D—main idea
2. B—supporting detail
3. A—meaning of word in context
4. B—author's purpose
5. C—author's tone
6. C—fact and opinion
7. B—inferences
8. D—summary

Bibliography

Johnson B: *The reading edge*, ed 4, New York, 2001, Houghton Mifflin.

VOCABULARY

Members of the health professions use specific medical terminology to ensure accurate, concise, and consistent communication among all persons involved in the provision of health care. In addition to the use of specific medical terms, many general vocabulary words are used in a health care context. It is essential that students planning to enter the health care field have a basic understanding of these general vocabulary words to ensure accurate communication in a professional setting.

The following list of vocabulary words includes a definition for each word and an example of the word used in a health care context. Careful study and review of these vocabulary words will help you begin your health profession studies with the ability to communicate in a professional manner.

HESI Hint • Being able to use a wide range of vocabulary skills correctly is considered by some experts to be the best measure of adult IQ.

Abrupt: Sudden.

Example: The nurse noticed an abrupt change in the patient's level of pain.

Abstain: To voluntarily refrain from something.

Example: The dental hygienist instructed the patient to abstain from smoking to improve his breath odor.

Access: A means to obtain entry or a means of approach.

Example: To administer medications into the patient's vein, the nurse must access the vein with a special needle.

Accountable: Responsible.

Example: Paramedics are accountable for maintaining up-to-date knowledge of resuscitation techniques.

Adhere: To hold fast or stick together.

Example: The tape must adhere to the patient's skin to hold the bandage in place.

Adverse: Undesired, possibly harmful.

Example: Vomiting is an adverse effect of many medications.

Affect: Appearance of observable emotions.

Example: The nurse observed that a depressed patient exhibited no obvious emotion and reported that the patient had a flat affect.

Annual: Occurring every year.

Example: The patient told the nurse that she had scheduled her annual mammogram, as she had been instructed.

Apply: To place, put on, or spread something.

Example: The physical therapist will apply a medication to the wound before covering the wound with a bandage.

Audible: Able to be heard.

Example: The respiratory therapist noticed that when the patient was having difficulty breathing, the therapist could hear an audible wheezing sound.

Bilateral: Present on two sides.

Example: The unlicensed assistive personnel reported to the nurse that the patient had bilateral weakness in the legs when walking.

Cast: Hard protective device applied to protect a broken bone while the bone heals.

Example: The nurse instructed the child that he could not go swimming while the cast was on his broken arm.

Cease: Come to an end or bring to an end.

Example: Because the patient's breathing had ceased, the paramedic began resuscitation measures.

Compensatory: Offsetting or making up for something.

Example: When the patient's blood pressure decreased, the paramedic noted that the heart rate increased, which the paramedic recognized as a compensatory action.

Complication: An undesired problem that is the result of some other event.

Example: The physician told the patient that loss of eyesight is a possible complication of eye surgery.

Comply: Do as directed.

Example: The nurse asked the patient to comply with the instructions for taking the medication.

Concave: Rounded inward.

Example: The dietician noticed that the patient was very thin, and the patient's abdomen appeared concave.

Concise: Brief, to the point.

Example: When teaching a patient, the nurse tried to be concise, so the instructions would be easy to remember.

Consistency: Degree of viscosity; how thick or thin a fluid is.

Example: The respiratory therapist noticed that the mucus the patient was coughing was of a thin, watery consistency.

Constrict: To draw together or become smaller.

Example: The nurse knows that the small blood vessels of the skin will constrict when ice is applied to the skin.

Contingent: Dependent.

Example: The hygienist told the patient that a healthy mouth is contingent on careful daily brushing and flossing.

Contour: Shape or outline of a shape.

Example: While bathing an overweight patient, the unlicensed assistive personnel noticed that the contour of the patient's abdomen was quite rounded.

Contract: To draw together, to reduce in size.

Example: The physical therapist exercises the patient's muscles so they contract and expand.

Contraindication: A reason why something is not advisable or why it should not be done.

Example: The patient's excessive bleeding was a contraindication for discharge from the hospital.

Defecate: Expel feces.

Example: The unlicensed assistive personnel helped the patient to the toilet when he needed to defecate.

Deficit: A deficiency or lack of something.

Example: The therapist explained that the patient will experience a fluid deficit if the patient continues to perspire heavily during exercise without drinking enough fluids.

Depress: Press downward.

Example: The nurse will depress the patient's skin to see if any swelling is present.

Depth: Downward measurement from a surface.

Example: The physician measures the depth of a wound by inserting a cotton swab into the wound.

Deteriorating: Worsening.

Example: The dental hygienist explains that the condition of the patient's gums is deteriorating, and treatment by the dentist is needed right away.

Device: Tool or piece of equipment.

Example: A thermometer is a device used to measure the patient's body temperature.

Diameter: The distance across the center of an object.

Example: When measuring a patient's blood pressure, the nurse knows that when the diameter of a blood vessel increases, the pressure in that blood vessel goes down.

Dilate: To enlarge or expand.

Example: When shining a light in the patient's eyes, the nurse looks to see if both pupils dilate in response to the light.

Dilute: To make a liquid less concentrated.

Example: So that the medication will be easier to swallow, the nurse uses fruit juice to dilute a foul-tasting drug.

Discrete: Distinct, separate.

Example: The paramedic observed several discrete bruise marks on the patient's body.

Distended: Enlarged or expanded from pressure.

Example: When a blood vessel is distended, it is easier for the laboratory technician to insert a needle to obtain a blood sample.

Elevate: To lift up or place in a higher position.

Example: The paramedic decided to elevate the head of the stretcher in order to help the patient breathe more easily.

Endogenous: Produced within the body.

Example: The nurse explained that endogenous insulin produced by the body's pancreas helps regulate the body's blood sugar levels.

Exacerbate: To make worse or more severe.

Example: The physical therapist recognized that too much exercise would exacerbate the patient's breathing difficulties.

Excess: More than what is needed or usual.

Example: The dietician explained that an excess consumption of caffeine may cause unpleasant effects such as feeling nervous and on edge.

Exogenous: Produced outside the body.

Example: The nurse explained that people with diabetes often need to receive exogenous forms of insulin because their bodies are unable to produce enough insulin.

Expand: To increase in size or amount.

Example: The unlicensed assistive personnel turns the patient frequently so that the size of the skin sore will not expand any further.

Exposure: Contact.

Example: The nurse taught the parents of a newborn to avoid exposure to people with severe infections.

External: Located outside the body.

Example: The unlicensed assistive personnel measured the amount of blood in the external drain after the patient's surgery.

Fatal: Resulting in death.

Example: The emergency medical technicians arrived too late to save any lives at the scene of a fatal car accident.

Fatigue: Extreme tiredness, exhaustion.

Example: The dietician explained to the patient that eating more iron-rich foods may help reduce feelings of fatigue.

Flaccid: Limp, lacking tone.

Example: After her stroke, the patient could not feed herself because her arms were flaccid.

Flushed: Reddened or ruddy appearance.

Example: The therapist observed that the patient's face was flushed after completing the exercises.

Gaping: Wide open.

Example: In the emergency room, the nurse observed a gaping wound when examining a gunshot victim.

Gender: Sex of an individual, as in male or female.

Example: Female gender places patients at higher risk for breast cancer.

Hydration: Maintenance of body fluid balance.

Example: The nurse explains that adequate hydration helps keep skin soft and supple.

Hygiene: Measures contributing to cleanliness and good health.

Example: The dental assistant teaches patients about good hygiene practices to maintain strong teeth.

Impaired: Diminished or lacking some usual quality or level.

Example: The paramedic stated that the patient's impaired speech was obvious in the way she slurred her words.

Impending: Likely to occur soon.

Example: The nurse observed the patient signing the consent form for the impending procedure.

Incidence: Occurrence.

Example: In recent years there has been an increased incidence of infections that do not respond to antibiotics.

Inflamed: Reddened, swollen, warm, and often tender.

Example: The nurse observed that the skin around the patient's wound was inflamed.

Ingest: To swallow for digestion.

Example: The paramedic may contact the poison control center when providing emergency care for a child who has ingested cleaning fluid.

Initiate: To begin or put into practice.

Example: The nurse decided to initiate safety measures to prevent injury because the patient was very weak.

Insidious: So gradual as to not become apparent for a long time.

Example: The physician explained that the cancer probably started years ago but had not been detected because its spread was so insidious.

Intact: In place, unharmed.

Example: The nurse observed that the bandage was intact after surgery.

Internal: Located within the body.

Example: The paramedic reported that the patient was unconscious because of internal bleeding.

Invasive: Inserting or entering into a body part.

Example: The laboratory technician is careful when obtaining blood samples, because this invasive procedure may cause problems such as infection or bruising.

Labile: Changing rapidly and often.

Example: Because the child's temperature was very labile, the nurse instructed the unlicensed assistive personnel to check the temperature frequently.

Latent: Present, but not active or visible.

Example: The latent infection produced symptoms only when the patient's condition was weakened from another illness.

Lethargic: Difficult to arouse.

Example: The unlicensed assistive personnel observed that the morning after a patient received a sleeping pill, the patient was too lethargic to eat breakfast.

Manifestation: An indication or sign of a condition.

Example: The dietician looked for manifestations of poor nutrition, such as excessive weight loss and poor skin condition.

Nutrient: Substance or ingredient that provides nourishment.

Example: The dietician explains that fruits and vegetables contain nutrients that reduce the risk of some cancers.

Occluded: Closed or obstructed.

Example: Because the patient's foot was cold and blue, the nurse reported that the patient's circulation to that foot was occluded.

Ominous: Significantly important and dangerous.

Example: After a patient sustained a head injury, the paramedic noted that the patient's breathing was irregular, which was an ominous sign that the patient's condition was worsening.

Ongoing: Continuous.

Example: The nurse instructed the patient that the treatment would be ongoing throughout the patient's entire hospital stay.

Oral: Given through or affecting the mouth.

Example: The unlicensed assistive personnel reminded the patient not to take any fluids orally because he was scheduled for surgery.

Overt: Obvious, easily observed.

Example: The overt symptoms of the disease included vomiting and diarrhea.

Parameter: A characteristic or constant factor.

Example: The dietician explained that the number of calories needed for energy is one of the important parameters of a healthy diet.

Paroxysmal: Beginning suddenly or abruptly.

Example: The respiratory therapist provided a breathing treatment to stop the patient's paroxysmal breathing difficulty.

Patent: Open.

Example: The nurse checked to see whether the intravenous needle was patent before giving the patient a medication.

Potent: Producing a strong effect.

Example: The medication was very potent, and it immediately relieved the patient's pain.

Potential: Capable of occurring or likely to occur.

Example: Because the patient was very weak, the therapist felt the patient had a high potential for falling.

Precaution: Preventive measure.

Example: The laboratory technician wore gloves as a precaution against blood contamination.

Precipitous: Rapid, uncontrolled.

Example: The paramedic assisted the pregnant woman during a precipitous delivery in her home.

Predispose: To make more susceptible or more likely to occur.

Example: The dietician explains that high dietary fat intake predisposes some persons to heart disease.

Preexisting: Already present.

Example: The nurse notified the physician that the patient has a preexisting condition that might lead to complications during the emergency surgery.

Primary: First or most significant.

Example: The patient's primary concern was when he could return to work after the operation.

Priority: Of great importance.

Example: The laboratory technician was gentle when inserting the needle because it is a high priority to ensure that the patient does not experience excessive pain and discomfort during the procedure.

Prognosis: The anticipated or expected course or outcome.

Example: The physician explained that with treatment the patient's prognosis was for a long and healthy life.

Rationale: The underlying reason.

Example: To make sure that the patient will follow the diet instructions, the dietician explains the rationale for the low-salt diet.

Recur: To occur again.

Example: To make sure that a tooth cavity does not recur, the dental hygienist instructs the patient to use toothpaste with fluoride regularly.

Restrict: To limit.

Example: The unlicensed assistive personnel removed the water pitcher from the room to assist the patient in following instructions to restrict the intake of fluids.

Retain: To hold or keep.

Example: The nurse administered a medication to prevent the patient from retaining excess body fluid, which might cause unpleasant swelling.

Site: Location.

Example: The nurse selected a site to start the patient's IV based on comfort for the patient.

Status: Condition.

Example: The paramedic recognized that the patient's status was unstable, which necessitated immediate transport to the nearest medical center.

Strict: Stringent, exact, complete.

Example: The nurse stressed that the patient must follow instructions to maintain strict bed rest to prevent further injury.

Supplement: To take in addition to or to complete.

Example: The dietician instructed the patient to supplement their diet with extra calcium tablets to help build strong bones.

Suppress: To stop or subdue.

Example: When the child's fever came down, the nurse checked to see if any medications had been given that would have suppressed the fever.

Symmetric (symmetrical): Being equal or the same in size, shape, and relative position.

Example: The paramedic observed that the movement of both sides of the patient's chest was symmetrical after the accident.

Symptom: An indication of a problem.

Example: The nurse recognized that the patient's weakness was a symptom of bleeding after surgery.

Untoward: Adverse or negative.

Example: The patient became very confused, which was an untoward effect of the medication received.

Urinate: Excrete or expel urine.

Example: The nurse instructed the patient to report any discomfort felt during urination.

Verbal: Spoken, using words.

Example: The paramedic called in a verbal report on the patient's condition to the emergency room nurse while transporting the patient to the hospital.

Vital: Essential.

Example: The paramedic knows that it is vital to learn what type of poison was taken when caring for a poisoning victim.

Void: Excrete, or expel urine.

Example: The patient was instructed to void into the container so the nurse could observe the appearance of the urine.

Volume: Amount of space occupied by a fluid.

Example: The nurse recorded the volume of cough syrup administered to the patient.

Sample Vocabulary Questions

1. What word meaning "once a year" fits best in the sentence?
   The _____ family reunion picnic was held at the Jones farm instead of the county park.
   A. regular
   B. annual
   C. biennial
   D. holiday

2. Select the word that means "an undesired problem that is the result of some other event."
   The complication of the surgery caused the patient to remain in the hospital to have an additional complement of testing procedures implemented.
   A. complication
   B. complement
   C. procedures
   D. implemented

3. Select the word that means "brief, to the point."
   The teacher's instructions were concise, so the student was able to complete the project in a reasonable period of time.
   A. instructions
   B. concise
   C. complete
   D. reasonable

4. Select the meaning of the underlined word in the sentence.
   The dog developed bilateral weakness in its hindquarters, so the veterinarian created a wheeled cart to help the dog walk.
   A. Present on two sides
   B. Available for exercise
   C. Affecting the left side
   D. Affecting the right side

5. Select the meaning of the underlined word in the sentence.
   The child developed a labile condition that worried the parents, so they brought the child to the doctor's office for a checkup.
   A. Fevered
   B. Volatile
   C. Stomach
   D. Vision

6. Select the correct definition of the underlined word.
   The gaping hole in the fence was an enticing lure for the curious toddler.
   A. Narrow
   B. Jagged
   C. Painted
   D. Wide open

7. Select the correct definition of the underlined word.
   The incidence of smoking has decreased in recent years because of the effectiveness of advertising campaigns.
   A. Prestige
   B. Glamour
   C. Occurrence
   D. Influence

8. Select the correct definition of the underlined word.
   The <u>symmetrical</u> nature of the artwork allowed it to be viewed from many angles.
   A. Measured from the center
   B. Colorful
   C. Equal on all sides
   D. Whimsical

9. Select the correct definition of the underlined word.
   The <u>verbal</u> instructions given by the instructor allowed the student to create an outstanding project.
   A. Written
   B. Detailed
   C. Oral
   D. Permissive

10. Select the correct definition of the underlined word.
   The doctor's <u>prognosis</u> gave the patient and his family reason to feel optimistic about the surgery.
   A. Instructions
   B. Estimate
   C. Behavior
   D. Outcome statement

Answers to Sample Vocabulary Questions

1. B—annual
2. A—complication
3. B—concise
4. A—Present on two sides
5. B—Volatile

6. D—Wide open
7. C—Occurrence
8. C—Equal on all sides
9. C—Oral
10. D—Outcome statement

GRAMMAR

In the United States, the ability to speak and write the English language using proper grammar is one sign of an educated individual. When people are sick and need information or care from individuals in the health professions, they expect healthcare workers to be professional and well educated individuals. It is therefore imperative that anyone in health care understand and use proper grammar.

Grammar varies a great deal from language to language. English as a second language (ESL) students have an added burden to becoming successful. For example, nursing research literature indicates that ESL nursing students are at greater risk for attrition and failure of the licensing examination. However, this burden can be overcome by learning proper grammar.

This chapter describes the parts of speech, important terms and their uses in grammar, commonly occurring grammatical errors, and suggestions for successful use of grammar.

Eight Parts of Speech

The eight parts of speech are nouns, pronouns, adjectives, verbs, adverbs, prepositions, conjunctions, and interjections.

NOUN

A noun is a word or group of words that names a person, place, thing, or idea.
Common Noun A common noun is the general, not the particular, name of a person, place, or thing (e.g., *nurse, hospital, syringe*).
Proper Noun A proper noun is the official name of a person, place, or thing (e.g., *Susan, Houston, St. Luke's Episcopal Hospital*). Proper nouns are capitalized.
Abstract Noun An abstract noun is the name of a quality or a general idea (e.g., *persistence, democracy*).
Collective Noun A collective noun is a noun that represents a group of persons, animals, or things (e.g., *family, flock, furniture*).

PRONOUN

A pronoun is a word that takes the place of a noun, another pronoun, or a group of words acting as a noun. The word or group of words to which a pronoun refers is called the *antecedent*.

The *students* wanted *their* test papers graded and returned to them in a timely manner.

The word *students* is the antecedent of the pronoun *their*.
Personal Pronoun A personal pronoun refers to a specific person, place, thing, or idea by indicating the person speaking (first person), the person or people spoken to (second person), or any other person, place, thing, or idea being talked about (third person).

Personal pronouns also express number in that they are either singular or plural.

We [first person plural] were going to ask *you* [second person singular] to give *them* [third person plural] a ride to the office.

Possessive Pronoun A possessive pronoun is a form of personal pronoun that shows possession or ownership.

That is *my* book.
That book is *mine*.
That is *his* book.
That book is *his*.

A possessive pronoun does not contain an apostrophe.

ADJECTIVE

An adjective is a word, phrase, or clause that modifies a noun (the *biology* book) or pronoun (*He* is nice.). It answers the question *what kind* (a *hard* test), *which one* (an *Evolve Reach* test), *how many* (*three* tests), or *how much* (*many* tests). Verbs, pronouns, and nouns can act as adjectives. Adjectives usually precede the noun or noun phrase that they modify—for example, *the absent-minded professor.*

Examples

Verbs: the *scowling* professor, the *worried* student, the *broken* pencil
Pronouns: *my* book, *your* class, *that* book, *this* class
Nouns: the *professor's* class, the *biology* class

VERB

A verb is a word or phrase that is used to express an action or a state of being. A verb is the critical element of a sentence. Verbs express time through a property that is called the *tense*. The three primary tenses are:

- Present—Mary *works*
- Past—Mary *worked*
- Future—Mary *will work*

Some verbs are known as "linking verbs" because they link, or join, the subject of the sentence to a noun, pronoun, or predicate adjective. A linking verb does not show action.

- The most commonly used linking verbs are forms of the verb *to be: am, is, are, was, were, being, been* (e.g., That man *is* my professor.).
- Linking verbs are sometimes verbs that relate to the five senses: *look, sound, smell, feel,* and *taste* (e.g., That exam *looks* difficult.).
- Sometimes linking verbs reflect a state of being: *appear, seem, become, grow, turn, prove,* and *remain* (e.g., The professor *seems* tired.).

> **HESI Hint** • The following are examples of proper and improper grammar related to verb usage:
>
> It is important that Vanessa send [**not** *sends*] her resume immediately.
> I wish I were [**not** *was*] that smart.
> If I were [**not** *was*] you, I'd leave now.

ADVERB

An adverb is a word, phrase, or clause that modifies a verb, an adjective, or another adverb.

Examples

Verb: The physician operates *quickly*.
Adjective: The nurse wears *very* colorful uniforms.
Another Adverb: The student scored *quite* badly on the test.

PREPOSITION

A preposition is a word that shows the relationship of a noun or pronoun to some other word in the sentence. A compound preposition is a preposition that is made up of more than one word. A prepositional phrase is a group of words that begins with a preposition and ends with a noun or a pronoun

BOX 4-1 *Commonly Used Prepositions*		
aboard	by	opposite
about	concerning	out
above	considering	outside
across	despite	over
after	down	past
against	during	pending
along	except	plus
amid	following	prior to
among	for	throughout
around	from	to
as	in	toward
at	including	under
barring	inside	underneath
before	into	unlike
behind	like	until
below	minus	up
beneath	near	upon
beside	of	with
between	off	within
beyond	on	without
but (except)	onto	

called the *object* of the proposition. Box 4-1 lists commonly used prepositions.

CONJUNCTION

A conjunction is a word that joins words, phrases, or clauses. Words that serve as *coordinating* conjunctions are *and, but, or, so, nor, for,* and *yet* (e.g., The nurse asked to work the early shift, *but* her request was denied.).

Correlative conjunctions work in pairs to join words or phrases (e.g., *Neither* the pharmacist *nor* her assistant could read the physician's handwriting.).

Sometimes conjunctions join two clauses or thoughts (e.g., While the nurse was away on vacation, the hospital flooded.). *While the nurse was away on vacation* is dependent on the rest of the sentence to complete its meaning.

INTERJECTION

An interjection is a word or phrase that expresses emotion or exclamation. It does not have any grammatical connection to the other words in the sentence (e.g., *Yikes*, that test was hard. *Whew*, that test was easy.).

Nine Important Terms to Understand

There are nine important terms to understand: clause, direct object, indirect object, phrase, predicate, predicate adjective, predicate nominative, sentence, and subject.

CLAUSE

A clause is a group of words that has a subject and a predicate.
Independent Clause An independent clause expresses a complete thought and can stand alone as a sentence (e.g., *The professor distributed the examinations as soon as the students were seated.*). *The professor distributed the examinations* expresses a complete thought and can stand alone as a sentence.
Dependent Clause A dependent clause does not express a complete thought and therefore cannot stand alone as a sentence. *As soon as the students were seated* does not express a complete thought. It needs the independent clause to complete the meaning and form the sentence.

DIRECT OBJECT

A direct object is the person or thing that is directly affected by the action of the verb. A direct object answers the question *what* or *whom* after a transitive verb.

> The students watched the professor distribute the examinations.
>
> *The professor* answers *whom* the students watched.

INDIRECT OBJECT

An indirect object is the person or thing that is indirectly affected by the action of the verb. A sentence can have an indirect object only if it has a direct object. An indirect object answers the question *to whom, for whom, to what,* or *for what* after an action verb.
    Indirect objects always come between the verb and the direct object.

> The professor gave his class the test results.

His class is the indirect object. It comes between the verb *(gave)* and the direct object *(test results)*, and it answers the question *to whom*.

PHRASE

A phrase is a group of two or more words that acts as a single part of speech in a sentence. A phrase can be used as a noun, an adjective, or an adverb. A phrase lacks a subject and a predicate.

PREDICATE

A predicate is the part of the sentence that tells what the subject does or what is done to the subject. It includes the verb and all the words that modify the verb.

PREDICATE ADJECTIVE

A predicate adjective is an adjective that follows a linking verb and helps to explain the subject.

> My professors are *wonderful*.

PREDICATE NOMINATIVE

A predicate nominative is a noun or pronoun that follows a linking verb and helps to explain the subject.

> Professors are *teachers*.

SENTENCE

A sentence is a group of words that expresses a complete thought. Every sentence has a subject and a predicate.

SUBJECT

A subject is a word, phrase, or clause that names whom or what the sentence is about.

Ten Common Grammatical Mistakes

SUBJECT-VERB AGREEMENT

A subject must agree with its verb in number. A singular subject requires a singular verb. Likewise, a plural subject requires a plural verb.

Incorrect: The nurses [plural noun] *was* [singular verb] in a hurry to get there.

Correct: The nurses [plural noun] *were* [plural verb] in a hurry to get there.

There are times when the subject-verb agreement can be tricky to determine.

When the Subject and Verb Are Separated

Find the subject and verb and make sure they agree.

Incorrect: The *question* that appears on all of the tests *are* inappropriate.

Correct: The *question* that appears on all of the tests *is* inappropriate.

Ignore any intervening phrases or clauses. Ignore words such as *including, along with, as well as, together with, besides, except,* and *plus.*

Example: The *dean*, along with his class, *is* going on the tour of the facility.

Example: The *deans*, along with their classes, *are* going on the tour.

When the Subject Is a Collective Noun

A collective noun is singular in form but plural in meaning. It is a noun that represents a group of persons, animals, or things (e.g., *family, audience, committee, board, faculty, herd, flock*).

If the group is acting as a single entity, use a singular verb.

Example: The *faculty agrees* to administer the test.

If the group is acting separately, use a plural verb.

Example: The *faculty are* not in agreement about which test to administer.

When the Subject Is a Compound Subject

Usually when the subject consists of two or more words that are connected by the word *and*, the subject is plural and calls for a plural verb.

Example: The *faculty* and the *students are* in the auditorium.

When the subject consists of two or more singular words that are connected by the words *or, either/or, neither/nor,* or *not only/but also*, the subject is singular and calls for a singular verb.

Example: Neither the *student* nor the *dean was* on time for class.

When the subject consists of singular and plural words that are connected by the words *or, either/or, neither/nor,* or *not only/but also*, choose a verb that agrees with the subject that is closest to the verb.

Example: Either the *students* or the *teaching assistant is* responsible.

COMMA IN A COMPOUND SENTENCE

A compound sentence is a sentence that has two or more independent clauses. Each independent clause has a subject and a predicate and can stand alone as a sentence. When two independent clauses are joined by a coordinating conjunction such as *and, but, or,* or *nor*, place a comma before the conjunction.

Example: The professor thought the test was too easy, *but* the students thought it was too hard.

RUN-ON SENTENCE

A run-on sentence occurs when two or more complete sentences are written as though they were one sentence.

Example: The professor thought the test was too easy the students thought it was too hard.

A comma splice is one kind of run-on sentence. It occurs when two independent clauses are joined by only a comma.

Example: The professor thought the test was too easy, the students thought it was too hard.

The problem can be solved by replacing the comma with a dash, a semicolon, or a colon, by adding a coordinating conjunction, or by making two separate sentences.

PRONOUN CASE

Is it correct to say, "It was *me*" or "It was *I*"; "It must be *they*" or "It must be *them*"?

Knowing which pronoun to use has to do with the pronoun's case. *Case* refers to the form of a noun or pronoun that indicates its relation to the other words in a sentence. There are three cases: *nominative, objective,* and *possessive*. The case of a personal pronoun depends on the pronoun's function in the sentence. The pronoun can function as a subject, a complement (predicate nominative, direct object, or indirect object), an object of a preposition, or a replacement for a possessive noun.

Examples—Pronoun Use

- When the pronoun is the subject
  - I studied for the examination.
  - *I* is the subject of the sentence. Therefore use the nominative form of the pronoun.

- When pronouns are the subject in a compound subject
    - Is it correct to say, *"**He and I** went to the conference"* or *"**Him and me** went to the conference"*?
    - Is it accurate to say, *"**John and me** worked through the night"* or *"**John and I** worked through the night"*?
    - Is it proper to say, *"**Her and Maria** liked the chocolate-covered toffee"* or *"**She and Maria** liked the chocolate-covered toffee"*?

Knowing which pronoun is accurate requires understanding how the pronoun is used in the sentence, so we know to use the nominative case. Therefore *He and I, I,* and *She* are the accurate forms of the pronouns.

> **HESI Hint** • When choosing a pronoun that is in a compound subject, sometimes it is helpful to say the sentence without the conjunction and the other subject. We would not say, *Him went to the conference* or *Me worked through the night* or *Her liked the chocolate-covered toffee*. We would, however, say, *He went to the conference* and *I worked through the night* and *She liked the chocolate-covered toffee*.

> **HESI Hint** • It is considered polite to place the pronoun *I* last in a series: *Luke, Jo, and I strive to do a good job*.

- When the pronoun is the object of the preposition

Susan gave the results of the test to them.

The pronoun *them* is the object of the preposition *to*. When the object of the preposition is a compound object as in *Susan gave the results of the test to **Jo and me***, the objective form of the pronoun is used.

- When the pronoun replaces a possessive noun

That desk is hers.

The possessive pronoun *hers* is used to replace a possessive noun. For example, suppose there is a desk that belongs to Holly. We would say,

That desk belongs to Holly. That is Holly's desk. That desk is Holly's. That desk is hers.

> **HESI Hint** • Do not use an apostrophe with a possessive pronoun. There are no such words as *her's* or *their's*.

COMMA IN A SERIES

Use a comma to separate three or more items in a series or list. A famous dedication makes the problem apparent: "To my parents, Ayn Rand and God." Because of the comma placement, it appears as though Ayn Rand and God are the parents. Place a comma between each item in the list and before the conjunction in order to avoid confusion.

Example: The nursing student took classes in English, biology, and chemistry.

UNCLEAR OR VAGUE PRONOUN REFERENCE

An unclear or vague pronoun reference makes a sentence confusing and difficult to understand.

Example: The teacher and the student knew that she was wrong.

Who was wrong: the teacher or the student? The meaning is unclear. Rewrite the sentence to avoid confusion.

Example: The teacher and the student knew that the *student* was wrong.

SENTENCE FRAGMENTS

Sentence fragments are incomplete sentences.

Example: While the students were taking the test.

The students were taking the test is a complete sentence. However, use of the word *while* turns it into a dependent clause. In order to make the fragment a sentence, it is necessary to supply an independent clause.

Example: While the students were taking the test, the professor walked around the classroom.

> **HESI Hint** • Other words that commonly introduce dependent clauses are *among, because, although,* and *however*.

MISPLACED MODIFIER

Misplaced modifiers are words or groups of words that are not located properly in relation to the words they modify.

Example: I fear my teaching assistant may have discarded the test I was grading in the trash can.

Was the test being graded in the trash can? The modifier *in the trash can* has been misplaced. The sentence should be rewritten so that the modifier is next to the word, phrase, or clause that it modifies.

Example: I fear the test I was grading may have been discarded in the trash can by my teaching assistant.

PRONOUNS THAT INDICATE POSSESSION

The possessive forms of personal pronouns have their own possessive forms, as shown in Box 4-2. Do not confuse these possessive pronouns with contractions that are similarly pronounced or spelled. Examples are shown in Table 4-1.

PREPOSITIONS AT THE END OF A SENTENCE

As a general rule, it is not very graceful to end a sentence with a preposition.

Example: Where in the world did that grammar rule come from?

Often an attempt to repair the error can result in a clumsy and awkward sentence.

Example: From where in the world did that grammar rule come?

BOX 4-2 *Possessive Personal Pronouns*

I	My	Mine
He	His	His
She	Her	Hers
We	Our	Ours
You	Your	Yours
They	Their	Theirs
It	Its	Its

TABLE 4-1 Common Possessive Pronouns and Similar Contractions

Possessive Pronoun	Contraction
Its (belonging to *it*)	It's (it is, it has)
Their (belonging to *them*)	They're (they are)
Whose (belonging to *whom*)	Who's (who is, who has)

Sometimes the sentence can be rewritten.

Example: Where in the world did that grammar rule originate?

Winston Churchill poked fun at the problem in response to those who objected to prepositions at the end of sentences: "This is the sort of English up with which I will not put."

Four Suggestions for Success

ELIMINATE CLICHÉS

Clichés are expression or ideas that have lost their originality or impact over time because of excessive use. Examples of clichés are *blind as a bat, dead as a doornail, flat as a pancake, raining cats and dogs, keep a stiff upper lip, let the cat out of the bag, sick as a dog, take the bull by the horns, under the weather, white as a sheet,* and *you can't judge a book by its cover.*

Clichés should be avoided whenever possible because they are old, tired, and overused. If tempted to use a cliché, endeavor to rephrase the idea.

ELIMINATE EUPHEMISMS

A euphemism is a mild, indirect, or vague term that has been substituted for one that is considered harsh, blunt, or offensive. In many instances euphemisms are used in a sympathetic manner in order to shield and protect. Some people refuse to refer to someone who has died as "dead." Instead, they say that the person has *passed away, gone to be with the Lord,* or *met their Maker.* Euphemisms should be eliminated, and we should try to speak and write more accurately and honestly using our own words whenever appropriate.

It is also essential to use accurate and anatomically correct language when referring to the body, a body part, or a bodily function. To do otherwise is unprofessional and tactless.

ELIMINATE SEXIST LANGUAGE

Sexist language refers to spoken or written styles that do not satisfactorily reflect the presence of women in our society. Such language can suggest a sexist attitude on the part of the speaker or writer. Some believe that making men the default option is degrading and patronizing to women. In general, it is no longer considered appropriate to use *he* or *him* when referring to a hypothetical person. This can be especially important in contexts that refer to, for example, a physician as *he* or the nurse as *she*. In order to avoid such stereotypes, try to use gender-neutral titles that do not specify a particular gender. For example, use *firefighter* instead of *fireman*, *mail carrier* instead of *mailman*, *ancestors* instead of *forefathers*, *chair* instead of *chairman*, *supervisor* instead of *foreman*, *police officer* instead of *policeman*, and so on. Do not use terms such as *female doctor* or *male nurse* unless identifying the gender is necessary or appropriate. Similarly, do not use phrases such as *doctors and their wives*; use *doctors and their spouses* instead. If the idea is true that language shapes our thought processes, then we would do well to eliminate these sexist forms from our language.

ELIMINATE PROFANITY AND INSENSITIVE LANGUAGE

We are all aware that obscene and insensitive language includes more than George Carlin's seven words that cannot be said on television. Anyone can be insulting and cruel using any type of vocabulary if that is his or her objective. What we say does make a difference. The nursery rhyme we learned in our youth, "Sticks and stones may break my bones, but words will never hurt me," is simply not true. Just ask anyone who has been on the receiving end of language that is patronizing or demeaning. Because language constantly changes, sometimes we can be offensive without even realizing that we have committee a blunder. In the age of an "anything goes" attitude for television, music lyrics, and political back-stabbing, it is hard to know exactly what

constitutes offensive language. Once it was considered polite to use the term *colored* for *Negro*. Then the term *Afro-American* became the acceptable expression. It changed again to the word *black*, and now the preferred expression is *African American*. We need to be sensitive to language that excludes or emphasizes a person or group of people with reference to their race, sexual orientation, age, gender, religion, or handicap. We would all do well to remember another adage from childhood: the Golden Rule. Its message is clear: respect the dignity of every human being, and treat others as you would like to be treated.

Fifteen Troublesome Word Pairs

AFFECT VS. EFFECT

Affect is normally used as a verb that means "to influence or to change." (The chemotherapy *affected* [changed] my daily routine.) As a noun, *affect* is an emotional response or disposition. (The troubled teenager with the flat *affect* [disposition] attempted suicide.)

Effect may be used as a noun or a verb. As a noun it means "result or outcome." (The chemotherapy had a strange *effect* [result] on me.) As a verb, it means "to bring about or accomplish." (As a result of the chemotherapy, I was able to *effect* [bring about] a number of changes in my life.)

AMONG VS. BETWEEN

Use *among* to show a relationship involving more than two persons or things being considered as a group (The professor will distribute the textbooks *among* the students in his class).

Use *between* to show a relationship involving two persons or things (I sit *between* Holly and Jo in class), to compare one person or thing with an entire group (What's the difference between this book and other grammar books?), or to compare more than two things in a group if each is considered individually (I can't decide *between* the chemistry class, the biology class, or the anatomy class).

AMOUNT VS. NUMBER

Amount is used when referring to things in bulk (The nurse had a huge *amount* of paperwork).

Number is used when referring to individual, countable units (The nurse had a *number* of charts to complete).

GOOD VS. WELL

Good is an adjective. Use *good* before nouns (He did a *good* job) and after linking verbs (She smells *good*) to modify the subject. *Well* is usually an adverb. When modifying a verb, use the adverb *well* (She plays softball *well*). *Well* is used as an adjective only when describing someone's health (She is getting *well*).

> **HESI Hint** • To say that you feel well implies that you are in good health. To say that you are good or that you feel good implies that you are in good spirits.

BAD VS. BADLY

Apply the same rule for *bad* and *badly* that applies to good and well. Use *bad* as an adjective before nouns (He is a *bad* teacher) and after linking verbs (That smells *bad*) to modify the subject. Use *badly* to modify an action verb (The student behaved *badly* in class).

> **HESI Hint** • Do not use *badly* when using verbs that have to do with the senses. Say, "You felt *bad*." To say, "You felt *badly*" implies that something was wrong with your sense of touch. Say, "The mountain air smells wonderful." To say, "The mountain air smells wonderfully" implies that the air has a sense of smell that is used in a wonderful manner.

BRING VS. TAKE

Bring conveys action toward the speaker—to carry from a distant place to a near place (Please *bring* your textbooks to class).

Take conveys action away from the speaker—to carry from a near place to a distant place (Please *take* your textbooks home).

CAN VS. MAY (COULD VS. MIGHT)

Can and *could* imply ability or power (I *can* make an A in that class). *May* and *might* imply permission (You *may* leave early) or possibility (I *may* leave early).

FARTHER VS. FURTHER

Farther refers to a measurable distance (The walk to class is much *farther* than I expected). *Further* refers to a figurative distance and means "to a greater degree" or "to a greater extent" (I will have to study *further* to make better grades). *Further* also means "moreover" (*Further/Furthermore*, let me tell you something) and "in addition to" (The student had nothing *further* to say).

FEWER VS. LESS

Fewer refers to number—things that can be counted or numbered—and is used with plural nouns (The professor has *fewer* students in his morning class than he has in his afternoon class).

Less refers to degree or amount—things in bulk or in the abstract—and is used with singular nouns (*Fewer* patients mean *less* work for the staff). *Less* is also used when referring to numeric or statistical terms. (It's *less* than 2 miles to school. He scored *less* than 90 on the test. She spent *less* than $400 for this class. I am *less* than 5 feet tall.)

HEAR VS. HERE

Hear is a verb meaning "to recognize sound by means of the ear" (Can you *hear* me now?). *Here* is most commonly used as an adverb meaning "at or in this place" (The test will be *here* tomorrow).

i.e. VS. e.g.

The abbreviation *i.e.* (that is) is often confused with *e.g.* (for example); *i.e.* specifies or explains (I love to study chemistry, *i.e.*, the science dealing with the composition and properties of matter), and *e.g.* gives an example. (I love to study chemistry, *e.g.*, chemical equations, atomic structure, and molar relationships.)

LEARN VS. TEACH

Learn means "to receive or acquire knowledge" (I am going to *learn* all that I can about nursing). *Teach* means "to give or impart knowledge" (I will *teach* you how to convert decimals to fractions).

LIE VS. LAY

Lie means "to recline or rest." The principal parts of the verb are *lie, lay, lain,* and *lying*. Forms of *lie* are never followed by a direct object.

Examples

- I *lie* down to rest.
- I *lay* down yesterday to rest.
- I had *lain* down to rest.
- I was *lying* on the sofa.

Lay means "to put or place." The principal parts of the verb are *lay, laid, laid,* and *laying*. Forms of *lay* are followed by a direct object.

Examples

- I *lay* the book on the table.
- I *laid* the book on the table yesterday.
- I have *laid* the book on the table before.
- I am *laying* the book on the table now.

> **HESI Hint** • To help determine whether the use of *lie* or *lay* is appropriate in a sentence, substitute the word in question with "place, placed, placing" (whichever is appropriate). If the substituted word makes sense, the equivalent form of *lay* is correct. If the sentence doesn't make sense with the substitution, the equivalent form of *lie* is correct.

WHICH VS. THAT

Which is used to introduce nonessential clauses, and *that* is used to introduce essential clauses. A nonessential clause adds information to the sentence but is not necessary to make the meaning of the sentence clear. Use commas to set off a nonessential clause (The hospital, *which flooded last July*, is down the street). An essential clause adds information to the sentence that is needed to make the sentence clear. Do not use commas to set off an essential clause (All of the nurses *that work in ICU* are dedicated to their jobs).

WHO VS. WHOM

Who and *whom* serve as interrogative pronouns and relative pronouns. An interrogative pronoun is one that is used to form questions, and a relative pronoun is one that relates groups of words to nouns or other pronouns.

Examples

- *Who* is getting an A in this class? (Interrogative)
- Susan is the one *who* is getting an A in this class. (Relative)
- To *whom* shall I give the textbook? (Interrogative)
- Susan, *whom* the professor favors, is very bright. (Relative)

Who and *whom* may be singular or plural.

Examples

- *Who* is getting an A in this class? (Singular)
- *Who* are the students getting As in this class? (Plural)
- *Whom* did you say is passing the class? (Singular)
- *Whom* did you say are passing the class? (Plural)

Who is the nominative case. Use it for subjects and predicate nominatives.

> **HESI Hint** • Use *who* or *whoever* if *he, she, they, I,* or *we* can be substituted in the *who* clause.

Who passed the chemistry test? *He/she/they/I* passed the chemistry test.

Whom is the objective case. Use it for direct objects, indirect objects, and objects of the prepositions.

> **HESI Hint** • Use *whom* or *whomever* if *him, her, them, me,* or *us* can be substituted as the object of the verb or as the object of the preposition in the *whom* clause.

To *whom* did the professor give the test? He gave the test to *him/her/them/me/us*.

Summary

Review this chapter and ask yourself whether your use of the English language reflects that of an educated individual. If so, congratulations! If not, study the content of this chapter, and your scores on the Evolve Reach Admission Assessment are likely to improve.

Sample Grammar Questions

1. Which word is used incorrectly in the following sentence?
   Will you learn me how to do origami?
   A. origami
   B. learn
   C. will
   D. me

2. Which word is used incorrectly in the following sentence?
   To who should the letter be addressed?
   A. who
   B. should
   C. letter
   D. addressed

3. Select the best word for the blank in the following sentence.
   He couldn't _____ the speaker's words because of the nearby airport noise.
   A. here
   B. hear
   C. comprehend
   D. understand

4. Select the correct phrase to fit in the blank in the following sentence.
   _____ went to the rock band concert last night.
   A. He and I
   B. He and me
   C. Him and I
   D. Him and me

5. Select the correct word for the blank in the following sentence.
   The members of the group _____ to be seated together.
   A. wanting
   B. want
   C. wants
   D. waiting

6. Select the correct word for the blank in the following sentence.
   The student completed the test _____.
   A. quickly
   B. quick
   C. quitely
   D. quite

7. Select the correct word(s) for the blank in the following sentence.
   The student thought the second test was _____ than the first test.
   A. harder
   B. more hard
   C. hardest
   D. most hardest

8. Select the correct word for the blank in the following sentence.
   The dog wagged _____ tail when the food dish was filled.
   A. its
   B. it's
   C. the
   D. one's

9. What word is best to substitute for the underlined words in the following sentence?
   <u>The boy</u> watched the lights in the house go off.
   A. Him
   B. He
   C. His
   D. They
10. What word is used incorrectly in this sentence?
   The six students in the class discussed the test results between themselves.
   A. discussed
   B. results
   C. between
   D. themselves

Answers to Sample Grammar Questions

1. B—*Learn* is incorrect. Correct word is *teach*.
2. A—*Who* is incorrect. Correct word is *whom*.
3. B—*Hear* means to recognize sound by means of the ear. *Here* is a site differentiation. C and D would fit in the sentence, but the reference to airport noise makes B the best choice.
4. A—Pronouns used as subjects should be in the nominative form. B, C, and D contain objective forms.
5. B—The subject of the sentence (members) is plural, so the verb must agree (B). C would be correct if *group* was the subject. A and D do not make sense in the sentence.
6. A—Adverbs usually end in *ly*. A is the adverbial form and modifies *completed* in the sentence. B is an adjective, modifying a noun. C is misspelled *(quietly)*. D does not make sense.
7. A—Two things are being compared, so the comparative form is used. The modifiers *more* and *most* are incorrect to use with the comparative form. The -est form is used when comparing more than two items, so C is incorrect for that reason, and D is incorrect for double reasons of only two comparisons and not using *most* with the adverb *hardest*.
8. A—*Its*, the possessive pronoun. B is the contraction for *it is*. Neither C nor D makes sense in the context.
9. B—The correct form of pronouns is important. *He* should be substituted for *The boy* in this sentence. A and C are objective forms and should not be used as the subject of a sentence. D is a plural pronoun and should not be used to replace a singular noun.
10. C—*Between* implies only two people. The correct word to use in the sentence would be *among*. A, B, and D are used correctly.

BIOLOGY

5

Biology is the scientific study of life. Members of the health professions naturally deal with biology, whether it requires knowing the structure of a cell, understanding how a molecule will react to a medication or treatment, or comprehending how certain organisms in the body function. Prospective students desiring to enter one of the health professions should have a basic knowledge of biology.

This chapter reviews the structure and reactions of cells and molecules. The concepts of cellular respiration, photosynthesis, cellular reproduction, and genetics are also presented.

Biology Basics

In biology there is a hierarchic system of organization. The system is most inclusive as kingdom and least as species. The order is as follows:

- Kingdom
- Phylum
- Class
- Order
- Family
- Genus
- Species

Most scientists agree that the core theme in biology today is the idea of evolution. Charles Darwin first introduced this notion in 1859 in his book *On the Origin of Species*. He proposed that current species arose from a process he called "descent with modification."

Science is a process. For an experiment to be performed, several steps must be taken.

- The first step is hypothesis. This is simply a statement or explanation of certain events or happenings.
- The second step is the experiment. This is a repeatable procedure of gathering data to support or refute the hypothesis.
- The final step in the scientific process is the conclusion.

Water

Water is the substance that makes life possible. The molecule itself is simply two hydrogen atoms covalently bonded to one oxygen atom. The most significant aspect of water is the polarity of its bonds.

It is the polar nature of water that allows for hydrogen bonding between molecules. This type of intermolecular bonding has several resulting benefits. The first of these is water's high specific heat.

The specific heat of a molecule is the amount of heat necessary to raise the temperature of 1 gram of that molecule by 1° Celsius. Water has a relatively high specific heat value, which allows water to resist shifts in temperature. One powerful benefit is the ability of oceans or large bodies of water to stabilize climates.

Hydrogen bonding also results in strong cohesive and adhesive properties. Cohesion is the ability of a molecule to stay bonded or attracted to another molecule of the same substance. A good example is how water tends to run together on a newly waxed car. Adhesion is the ability of water to bond to or attract other molecules or substances. When water is sprayed on a wall, some of it sticks to the wall. That is adhesion.

When water freezes it forms a lattice, which actually causes the molecules to spread apart, resulting in the phenomenon of floating. Most molecules, when they are in the solid form, do not float on the liquid form of the substance. If ice did not float, lakes would freeze from the bottom to the top. Life could not exist as we know it.

The polarity of water also allows it to act as a versatile solvent. Water can be used to dissolve a number of different substances.

Biologic Molecules

There are multitudes of molecules that are significant to biology. The most important of these are carbohydrates, lipids, proteins, and nucleic acids.

CARBOHYDRATES

Carbohydrates are generally long chains, or polymers, of sugars. They have many functions and serve many different purposes. The most important of these are storage, structure, and energy.

LIPIDS

Lipids are better known as fats, but specifically are fatty acids, phospholipids, and steroids.

Fatty Acids Fatty acids vary greatly but simply are grouped into two categories: saturated and unsaturated. Saturated fats contain no double bonds in their hydrocarbon tail. Conversely, unsaturated fats have one or more double bonds. As a result, saturated fats are solid whereas unsaturated fats are liquid at room temperature. Saturated fats are those the general public considers detrimental, and cardiovascular problems are likely with diets that contain high quantities of saturated fats.

Phospholipids Phospholipids consist of two fatty acids of varying length bonded to a phosphate group. The phosphate group is charged and therefore polar, whereas the hydrocarbon tail of the fatty acids is nonpolar. This quality is particularly important in the function of cellular membranes. The molecules combine in a way that creates a barrier that protects the cell.

Steroids The last of the lipids are steroids. They are a component of membranes, but, more important, many are precursors to significant hormones.

PROTEINS

Proteins are the most significant contributor to cellular function. They are polymers of 20 molecules called *amino acids*. Complex and consisting of several structure types, proteins are the largest of the biological molecules. Enzymes are particular types of proteins that act to catalyze different reactions or processes. Nearly all cellular function is catalyzed by some type of enzyme.

NUCLEIC ACIDS

Nucleic acids are components of the molecules of inheritance. Deoxyribonucleic acid (DNA) is a unique molecule specific to a particular organism and contains the code that is necessary for replication. Ribonucleic acid (RNA) is used in transfer and as a messenger, in most species, of the genetic code.

Metabolism

Metabolism is the sum of all chemical reactions that occur in an organism. In a cell, reactions take place in a series of steps called *metabolic pathways*, progressing from a standpoint of high energy to low energy. All of the reactions are catalyzed by the use of enzymes.

The Cell

The cell is the fundamental unit of biology. There are two types of cells: prokaryotic and eukaryotic cells. Cells consist of many components, most of which are referred to as *organelles*.

Prokaryotic cells are those containing no defined nucleus and a series of organelles that carry out the functions of the cell as directed by the nucleus. Eukaryotic cells have a membrane-enclosed nucleus and a series of organelles that carry out the functions of the cell as directed by the nucleus. The eukaryotic cell is the more complex of the two cell types.

There are several different organelles functioning in a cell at a given time; only the major ones are considered here.

NUCLEUS

The first of the organelles is the nucleus, which contains the DNA of the cell in organized masses called *chromosomes*. Chromosomes contain all the material for the regeneration of the cell as well as all instructions for the function of the cell. Every organism has a characteristic number of chromosomes specific to the particular species.

RIBOSOMES

Ribosomes are organelles that read the RNA produced in the nucleus and translate the genetic instructions to produce proteins. Cells having a high rate of protein synthesis generally have a large number of ribosomes. There are two locations ribosomes can be found. Bound ribosomes are those found attached to the endoplasmic reticulum (ER), and free ribosomes are those found in the cytoplasm. The two types are interchangeable and have identical structures, although they have slightly different roles.

ENDOPLASMIC RETICULUM

The ER is a membranous organelle found attached to the nuclear membrane and consists of two continuous parts. Through an electron microscope, it is clear that part of the membranous system is covered with ribosomes. This section of the ER is referred to as *rough ER*, and it is responsible for protein synthesis and membrane production. The other section of the ER lacks ribosomes and is referred to as *smooth ER*. It functions in detoxification and metabolism of multiple molecules.

GOLGI APPARATUS

Inside the cell is a packaging, processing, and shipping organelle that is called the *Golgi apparatus*. The Golgi apparatus functions to transport materials from the ER throughout the cell.

LYSOSOMES

Intracellular digestion takes place in lysosomes. Packed with hydrolytic enzymes, the lysosomes can hydrolyze proteins, fats, sugars, and nucleic acids.

VACUOLES

Vacuoles are membrane-enclosed structures that have various functions depending on cell type. Many cells, through a process called *phagocytosis*, uptake food through the cell membrane, creating a food vacuole. Plant cells have a central vacuole that functions in storage, waste disposal, protection, and hydrolysis.

MITOCHONDRIA AND CHLOROPLASTS

There are two distinct organelles that produce cell energy: the mitochondrion and the chloroplast. Mitochondria are found in most eukaryotic cells and are the site of respiration. Chloroplasts are found in plants and are the site of photosynthesis.

CELLULAR MEMBRANE

The cellular membrane is the most important component of the cell, contributing to protection, communication, and the passage of substances into and out of the cell. The cell membrane itself consists of a bilayer of phospholipids with proteins, cholesterol, and glycoproteins peppered throughout. Because phospholipids are amphipathic molecules, this bilayer creates a hydrophobic region between the two layers of lipids, making it selectively permeable. Many of the proteins, which pass completely through the membrane, act as transport highways for molecular movement into and out of the cell.

Cellular Respiration

There are two catabolic pathways that lead to cellular energy production. As a simple combustion reaction, cellular respiration produces far more energy than does its anaerobic counterpart, fermentation.

$$C_6H_{12}O_6 + 6O_2 \rightarrow 6CO_2 + 6H_2O$$

This balanced equation is the simplified chemistry behind respiration. The process itself actually occurs in a series of three complex steps that are simplified for our purposes.

There is one molecule that is used as the currency of the cell: adenosine triphosphate (ATP). Another compound that acts as a reducing agent and is a vehicle of stored energy is reduced nicotinamide adenine dinucleotide (NADH). This molecule is used as a precursor to produce greater amounts of ATP in the final steps of respiration.

The first step is the conversion of glucose to pyruvate in a process called *glycolysis*. It takes place in the cytosol of the cell and produces two molecules of ATP, two molecules of pyruvate, and two molecules of NADH.

In step two, the pyruvate is transported into a mitochondrion and used in the first of a series of reactions called the *Krebs cycle*. This cycle takes place in the matrix of the mitochondria, and for a single consumed glucose molecule, two ATP molecules, six molecules of carbon dioxide, and six NADH molecules are produced.

The third step begins with the oxidation of the NADH molecules to produce oxygen and finally to produce water in a series of steps called the *electron transport chain*. The energy harvest here is remarkable. For every glucose molecule, 28 to 32 ATP molecules can be produced.

This conversion results in overall ATP production numbers of 32 to 36 ATP molecules for every glucose molecule consumed.

Photosynthesis

In the previous section the harvesting of energy by the cell was discussed. But where did that energy originate? It began with a glucose molecule and resulted in a large production of energy in the form of ATP. A precursor to the glucose molecule is produced in a process called *photosynthesis*.

The chemical reaction representing this process is simply the reverse of cellular respiration.

$$6CO_2 + 6H_2O + \text{Light energy} \rightarrow C_6H_{12}O_6 + 6O_2$$

The only notable difference is the addition of light energy on the reactant side of the equation. Just as glucose is used to produce energy, so too must energy be used to produce glucose.

Photosynthesis is not as simple a process as it looks from the chemical equation. In fact, it consists of two different stages: the light reactions and the Calvin cycle. The light reactions are those that convert solar energy to chemical energy. The cell accomplishes the production of ATP by absorbing light and using that energy to split a water molecule and transfer the electron, thus creating NADPH and producing ATP. These molecules are then used in the Calvin cycle to produce sugar.

The sugar produced is polymerized and stored as a polymer of glucose. These sugars are consumed by organisms or by the plant itself to produce energy by cellular respiration.

Cellular Reproduction

Cells reproduce by three different processes, all of which fall into two categories: sexual and asexual reproduction.

ASEXUAL REPRODUCTION

There are two types of asexual reproduction. The first involves bacterial cells and is referred to as *binary fission*. In this process, the chromosome binds to the plasma membrane, where it replicates. Then as the cell grows, it pinches in two, producing two identical cells.

Another type of asexual reproduction is called *mitosis*. This process of cell division occurs in five stages before pinching in two in a process called *cytokinesis*. The five stages are prophase, prometaphase, metaphase, anaphase, and telophase.

During prophase, the chromosomes are visibly separate, and each duplicated chromosome has two noticeable sister chromatids. In prometaphase, the nuclear envelope begins to disappear, and the chromosomes begin to attach to the spindle that is forming along the axis of the cell. Metaphase follows, with all the chromosomes aligning along what is called the *metaphase plate*, or the center of the cell. Anaphase begins when chromosomes start to separate. In this phase the chromatids are considered separate chromosomes. The final phase is telophase. Here chromosomes gather on either side of the now separating cell. This is the end of mitosis.

The second process associated with cell division is cytokinesis. During this phase, which is separate

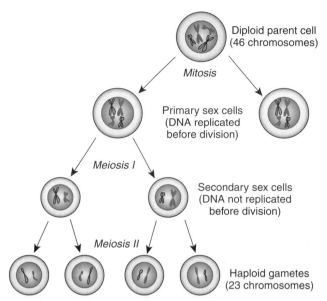

FIGURE 5-1 Two stages of meiosis: meiosis I and meiosis II. (From Thibodeau GA, Patton KT: *Anatomy and physiology*, ed 6, St Louis, 2007, Mosby.)

from the phases of mitosis, the cell pinches in two, forming two separate identical cells.

SEXUAL REPRODUCTION

Sexual reproduction is different from asexual reproduction. In asexual reproduction, the offspring originates from a single cell, yielding all produced cells to be identical. In sexual reproduction, two cells contribute genetic material to the daughter cells, resulting in significantly greater variation. These two cells find and fertilize each other randomly, making it virtually impossible for cells to be alike.

The process that determines how reproductive cells divide in a sexually reproducing organism is called *meiosis*. Meiosis consists of two distinct stages, meiosis one and meiosis two, resulting in four daughter cells (Figure 5-1). Each of these daughter cells contains half as many chromosomes as the parent. Preceding these events is a period called *interphase*. It is during interphase that the chromosomes are duplicated and the cell prepares for division.

The first stage of meiosis consists of four phases: prophase I, metaphase I, anaphase I, and telophase I and cytokinesis. The significant differences between meiosis and mitosis occur in prophase I. During this phase, nonsister chromatids of homologous chromosomes cross at numerous locations. Small sections of DNA are transferred between these chromosomes, resulting in increased genetic variation. The remaining three phases are the same as those in mitosis, with the exception that the chromosome pairs separate, not the chromosomes themselves.

After the first cytokinesis, meiosis two begins. Here, all four stages, identical to those of mitosis, occur. The resulting four cells have half as many chromosomes as the parent cell.

Genetics

Using garden peas, Gregor Mendel discovered the basic principles of genetics. By careful experimentation, he was able to determine that the observable traits in peas were passed from one generation to the next.

From Mendel's studies, scientists have found that for every trait expressed in a sexually reproducing organism, there are at least two alternative versions of a gene, called *alleles*. For simple traits, the versions can be one of two types: dominant or recessive. If both of the alleles are the same type, the organism is said to be *homozygous* for that trait. If they are different types, the organism is said to be *heterozygous*.

> **HESI Hint** • If an allele is dominant for a particular trait, the letter chosen to represent that allele is capitalized. If the allele is recessive, then the letter is lowercased. If a dominant allele is present, then the phenotype expressed will be the dominant. The only way a recessive trait will be expressed is if both alleles are recessive.

By use of a device called a *Punnett square*, it is possible to predict genotype (the combination of alleles) and phenotype (what traits will be expressed) of the offspring of sexual reproduction. Alleles are placed one per column for one gene and one per row for the other gene.

In the example in Figure 5-2 a homozygous dominant is crossed with a heterozygous organism for the same trait. Note that all progeny will express dominance for this trait.

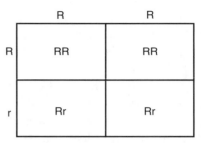

FIGURE 5-2   Punnett square depicting the cross between a homozygous dominant and a heterozygous organism.

In the example in Figure 5-3, three of the possible combinations will be dominant, and one will be recessive for this trait.

The Punnett square can be used to cross any number of different traits simultaneously. With these data, a probability of phenotypes that will be produced can be determined. However, the more traits desired, the more complex the cross.

Not all genes express themselves according to these simple rules, but they are the basis for all genetic understanding. There are many other methods of genetic expression. A few of these include multiple alleles, pleiotropy, epistasis, and polygenic inheritance.

Because genetics is the study of heredity, many human disorders can be detected by studying a person's chromosomes or by creating a pedigree. A pedigree is a family tree that traces the occurrence of a certain trait through several generations. A pedigree is useful in understanding the genetic past as well as the possible future.

DNA

DNA is the genetic material of a cell and is the vehicle of inheritance. In 1953, Watson and Crick described the structure of DNA. They described

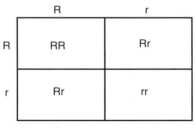

FIGURE 5-3   Punnett square depicting three possible dominant combinations.

a double helical structure that contains the four nitrogenous bases adenine, thymine, guanine, and cytosine.

Each base forms hydrogen bonds with another base on the complementary strand. The bases have a specific bonding pattern. Adenine bonds with thymine, and guanine bonds with cytosine. Because of this method of bonding, the strands can be replicated, producing identical strands of DNA. During replication, the strands are separated. Then, with the help of several enzymes, new complementary strands to each of the two original strands are created. This produces two new double-stranded segments of DNA identical to the original.

Each gene along a strand of DNA is a template for protein synthesis. This production begins with a process called *transcription*. In this process an RNA strand, complementary to the original strand of DNA, is produced. The piece of genetic material produced is called *messenger RNA* (mRNA). The RNA strand has nitrogenous bases identical to those in DNA with the exception of uracil, which is substituted for thymine.

mRNA functions as a messenger from the original DNA helix in the nucleus to the ribosomes in the cytosol or on the rough ER. Here, the ribosome acts as the site of translation. The mRNA slides through the ribosome. Every group of three bases along the stretch of RNA is called a *codon*, and each of these codes for a specific amino acid. The anticodon is located on a unit called *transfer RNA* (tRNA), which carries a specific amino acid. It binds to the ribosome when its codon is sliding through the ribosome. Remember that a protein is a polymer of amino acids, and multiple tRNA molecules bind in order and are released by the ribosome. Each amino acid is bonded together and released by the preceding tRNA molecule, creating an elongated chain of amino acids. Eventually the chain is ended at what is called a *stop codon*. At this point the chain is released into the cytoplasm, and the protein folds onto itself and forms its complete conformation.

By dictating what is produced in translation through transcription, the DNA in the nucleus has control over everything taking place in the cell. The proteins that are produced will perform all the different cellular functions required for the cell's survival.

Sample Biology Questions

1. What is the most important characteristic of water?
   A. Polarity of hydrogen bonding
   B. Polarity of the hydrogen-oxygen bonds
   C. High specific heat
   D. Versatile solvent
2. Which of the following biologic macromolecules are most important to the cellular membrane?
   A. Steroids
   B. Proteins
   C. Carbohydrates
   D. Phospholipids
3. What cellular organelle is the site of the catabolic pathway leading to cellular energy production?
   A. Mitochondrion
   B. Chloroplast
   C. Smooth ER
   D. Rough ER
4. What type of cellular reproduction do bacteria undergo?
   A. Mitosis
   B. Meiosis
   C. Binary fission
   D. Cellular division

5. What is the probability that a recessive trait would be expressed in offspring if two parents who are both heterozygous for the desired trait were crossed?
    A. 100%
    B. 75%
    C. 50%
    D. 25%
6. In which organelle does transcription begin?
    A. Ribosome
    B. Nucleus
    C. mRNA
    D. Cytoplasm

Answers to Sample Biology Questions

1. B—The most important characteristic of water is the polarity of its bonds. The results of the polarity are hydrogen bonding, a high specific heat value, and its versatile solvent properties.
2. D—The cellular membrane is able to function as a barrier protecting the cell because of the polarity of the phospholipid. Phospholipids are the key component that makes the membrane possible. Steroids, membrane proteins, and carbohydrates aid in the function of the membrane, but they are not responsible for its creation and well-being.
3. A—A catabolic pathway is one that breaks down molecules to produce energy. The organelle responsible for this is the mitochondrion. The chloroplast acts to harvest solar energy to store its chemical energy. The two forms of ER function to produce transport vesicles and proteins.

4. C—Bacteria are single-celled organisms that are not complex. They undergo a simple process of division called *binary fission*.
5. D—The second Punnett square in the section on genetics is a cross of the two parents who are heterozygous for the same trait. As you can see, there is a one in four (or 25%) chance that the recessive trait will be expressed. Remember that for the recessive trait to be expressed, both alleles must be recessive. If either is dominant, then the dominant will be expressed.
6. C—Transcription begins with the reading of the DNA in a cell to produce a complementary strand of mRNA. The DNA of the cell is located in the nucleus. Therefore the beginning of transcription takes place in the nucleus. The ribosome is the site of translation. Cytoplasm is the semitransparent, gelatinous fluid that is present in cells.

6

CHEMISTRY

Chemistry is a part of our everyday lives. Almost three quarters of the objective information in a client's record consists of laboratory data derived from chemical analytical testing. Laboratory tests play an important role in the detection, identification, and management of most diseases. The client's evaluation, diagnosis, treatment, care, and prognosis are based on chemical information from laboratory tests that involve traditional technologies and/or techniques involving chemistry. A sound, basic knowledge of chemistry enables the health care professional to reduce risk and deliver safe, high-quality care.

Students in the health professions need a basic understanding of both organic and inorganic chemistry. This chapter reviews chemistry from the simplest substances—that is, atoms and elements—to the more complex compounds existing in the three states of matter. Chemical bonding, molar relationships, stoichiometry, chemical reactions, and acids and bases are also presented.

Describing Matter

In chemistry, three states of matter are emphasized: solid, liquid, and gas. A solid is matter that has definite shape and volume. Both liquids and gases are matter that is fluid and takes the shape of its container. Unlike solids and liquids, the volume of gases will change drastically with changes in temperature and pressure.

There are two types of mixtures: homogeneous and heterogeneous. Homogeneous mixtures are those with uniform density throughout and no distinguishable components. Mixtures in which components are readily distinguished are heterogeneous.

It is important to understand the differences between chemical and physical changes. A physical change is one in which no change has been made to the chemical composition of the substance.

> **HESI Hint** • A good example would be the cutting of a cake. A chemical change is one in which the substance is changed by the breaking and reforming of bonds to create a new and different substance. The spoiling of an egg is a good example.

Chemical Equations and Reactions

An element is the simplest of substances and is represented by a specific letter or combination of letters. Compounds are combinations of elements in whole number ratios. All of the known elements can be found on the periodic table.

CHEMICAL EQUATIONS

Chemical equations are simply recipes. Ingredients, called *reactants*, react to produce a desired result, called *products*. Equations are written in the following manner:

$$\text{Reactants} \rightarrow \text{Products}$$

An example is the reaction of aqueous silver nitrate and aqueous potassium chloride to produce solid silver chloride and aqueous potassium nitrate.

$$AgNO_3 \text{ (aq)} + KCl \text{ (aq)} \rightarrow AgCl \text{ (s)} + KNO_3 \text{ (aq)}$$

The Law of Conservation of Mass states that mass cannot be created or destroyed during a chemical reaction. Therefore, once the reactants have been written and the products predicted, the equation must be balanced. The same number of each element must be represented on both sides of the equation.

CHEMICAL REACTIONS

A chemical reaction is the breaking of bonds and the reforming of new bonds to create new chemical compounds with different chemical formulas and different chemical properties. There are five main types of chemical reactions: synthesis, decomposition, combustion, single replacement, and double replacement.

In a synthesis reaction, two elements combine to form a product. Decomposition is the breaking of a compound into component parts. A combustion reaction is the reaction of a compound or element with oxygen. In the combustion of a hydrocarbon, the products are CO_2 and H_2O.

$$2C_2H_6 \text{ (g)} + 7O_2 \text{ (g)} \rightarrow 4CO_2 \text{ (g)} + 6H_2O \text{ (g)}$$

Replacement reactions involve ionic compounds, and whether the reaction will take place is based on the activity of the metals involved. Single replacement reactions consist of a more active metal reacting with an ionic compound containing a less active metal to produce a new compound. A good example is the reaction of copper wire with aqueous silver nitrate.

$$2Cu \text{ (s)} + 2AgNO_3 \text{ (aq)} \rightarrow 2Ag \text{ (s)} + Cu(NO_3)_2 \text{ (aq)}$$

Double replacement reactions involve two ionic compounds. The positive ion from one compound combines with the negative ion of the other compound. The result is two new ionic compounds that have "switched partners." The earlier example of the reaction of silver nitrate and potassium chloride is a good representation of double replacement.

$$AgNO_3 \text{ (aq)} + KCl \text{ (aq)} \rightarrow AgCl \text{ (s)} + KNO_3 \text{ (aq)}$$

Periodic Table

Elements are arranged according to their chemical properties on the periodic table (Figure 6-1). Although there are many trends represented, the

1	2	3	4	5	6	7	8	9	10	11	12	13	14	15	16	17	18
1 H 1.008																	2 He 4.002
3 Li 6.941	4 Be 9.012											5 B 10.811	6 C 12.011	7 N 14.007	8 O 15.999	9 F 18.998	10 Ne 20.180
11 Na 22.990	12 Mg 24.305											13 Al 26.982	14 Si 28.086	15 P 30.974	16 S 32.066	17 Cl 35.452	18 Ar 39.948
19 K 39.098	20 Ca 40.078	21 Sc 44.956	22 Ti 47.867	23 V 50.942	24 Cr 51.996	25 Mn 54.931	26 Fe 55.845	27 Co 58.933	28 Ni 58.963	29 Cu 63.546	30 Zn 65.39	31 Ga 69.723	32 Ge 72.61	33 As 74.922	34 Se 78.96	35 Br 79.904	36 Kr 83.80
37 Rb 85.468	38 Sr 87.62	39 Y 88.906	40 Zr 91.224	41 Nb 92.906	42 Mo 95.94	43 Tc (98)	44 Ru 101.07	45 Rh 102.906	46 Pd 106.42	47 Ag 107.868	48 Cd 112.411	49 In 114.818	50 Sn 118.710	51 Sb 121.760	52 Te 127.60	53 I 126.904	54 Xe 131.29
55 Cs 132.905	56 Ba 137.327	57 La 138.905	72 Hf 178.49	73 Ta 180.948	74 W 183.84	75 Re 186.207	76 Os 190.23	77 Ir 192.217	78 Pt 195.08	79 Au 196.967	80 Hg 200.59	81 Ti 204.383	82 Pb 207.2	83 Bi 208.980	84 Po (209)	85 At (210)	86 Rn (222)
87 Fr (223)	88 Ra 226.025	89 Ac 227.028	104 Unq (261)	105 Unp (262)	106 Unh (263)	107 Uns (262)	108 Uno (265)	109 Une (266)	110 Uun (269)								

58 Ce 140.115	59 Pr 140.907	60 Nd 144.24	61 Pm (145)	62 Sm 150.36	63 Eu 151.965	64 Gd 157.25	65 Tb 158.925	66 Dy 162.50	67 Ho 164.930	68 Er 167.26	69 Tm 168.939	70 Yb 173.04	71 Lu 174.967
90 Th 232.038	91 Pa 231.036	92 U 238.029	93 Np 237.048	94 Pu (244)	95 Am (243)	96 Cm (247)	97 Bk (247)	98 Cf (251)	99 Es (252)	100 Fm (257)	101 Md (258)	102 No (259)	103 Lr (260)

FIGURE 6-1   Periodic table of elements. (From Thibodeau GA, Patton KT: *Anatomy and physiology*, ed 6, St Louis, 2007, Mosby.)

most important is atomic number. It represents the number of protons a given element contains.

Each element also has associated with it an atomic mass. An element's atomic mass is an average of the masses of each of its isotopes as they occur in nature. By subtracting the atomic number from the mass number of an element, it is possible to calculate the number of neutrons contained by a given isotope of a certain element.

The groups (columns) and periods (rows) also have significance. It is possible to predict with accuracy the charge of an atom of certain elements when as an ion dissolved in solution or as an ion in a compound based on its location on the periodic table. Generally group IA has a +1 charge, group IIA a +2 charge, and group IIIA a +3 charge. The negative charges are as follows: group VA has −3, group VIA has −2, group VIIA has −1, and the noble gases have no charge; they remain neutral in nearly all applications.

Atomic Structure

The atom consists of three component parts: protons, neutrons, and electrons (Figure 6-2). Protons have a positive charge, electrons have a negative charge, and neutrons have no charge. Protons and

neutrons have approximately the same mass. Relative to the proton, the mass of an electron is 1840 times less. The number of protons in an element is its atomic number. The sum of the protons and neutrons in an atom is called the *mass number*.

> **HESI Hint** • It is important to note that the nucleus (dense center of the atom) contains the protons and the neutrons, whereas the electrons are located in orbitals (clouds) surrounding the nucleus. The majority of the volume of an atom is empty space

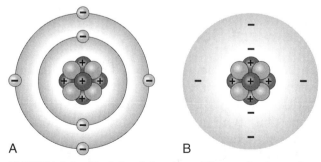

FIGURE 6-2   Models of the atom. The nucleus consists of protons (+) and neutrons at the core. Electrons inhabit outer regions called electron shells or energy levels (A) or (B) clouds. (From Thibodeau GA, Patton KT: *Anatomy and physiology*, ed 6, St Louis, 2007, Mosby.)

Nuclear Chemistry

Chemical and nuclear reactions are quite different. In chemical reactions, atoms try to reach stable electron configurations. Nuclear reactions are those that take place in the nucleus, to obtain stable nuclear configurations.

Radioactivity is the word used to describe the emission of particles from an unstable nucleus. The particles that are emitted are referred to as *radiation*. There are three types of radiation covered in general chemistry: alpha, beta, and gamma.

ALPHA RADIATION

Alpha radiation is the emission of helium ions. These particles contain two protons and two neutrons, causing them to have a charge of +2. However, it is common to omit the fact that these particles are charged. Penetration from alpha particles can generally be stopped by a piece of paper.

BETA RADIATION

Beta radiation is a product of the decomposition of a neutron. It is actually composed of high-energy, high-speed electrons. These particles are negatively charged and have virtually no mass. Beta particles can be stopped by aluminum foil.

GAMMA RADIATION

Gamma radiation is high-energy electromagnetic radiation. Gamma rays lack charge and mass. This form of radiation can be stopped by several feet of concrete or several inches of lead.

Chemical Bonding

There are two main types of chemical bonding: covalent and ionic. An ionic bond is an electrostatic attraction between two oppositely charged ions. This type of bond is generally formed between metals and nonmetals.

A single covalent bond is formed when two atoms share a pair of electrons. A double covalent bond is formed when two electron pairs are shared (Figure 6-3), and a triple covalent bond is formed when three electron pairs are shared. The covalent bond

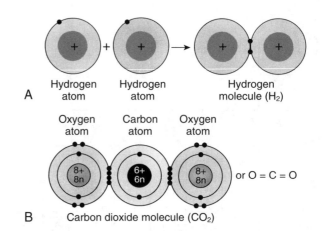

FIGURE 6-3 Types of covalent bonds. A, A single covalent bond forms by the sharing of one electron pair between two atoms of hydrogen, resulting in a molecule of hydrogen gas. **B,** A double covalent bond (double bond) forms by the sharing of two pairs of electrons between two atoms. In this case two double bonds form: one between carbon and each of the two oxygen atoms. (From Thibodeau GA, Patton KT: *Anatomy and physiology,* ed 6, St Louis, 2007, Mosby.)

is the strongest of any type of chemical bond. It is generally formed between nonmetals.

In a covalently bonded compound, if the electrons in the bond are shared equally, then the bond is nonpolar. However, not all elements share electrons equally within a bond. When this occurs, a polar covalent bond is the result. Polarity is based on the difference in electronegativity values for the elements involved in the bond. The greater the difference, the more polar the bond will be. There are other types of attractions between particles called *intermolecular forces*. These forces are hydrogen bonding, dipole interactions, and dispersion forces. The last two forces are also called *van der Waals forces*.

HYDROGEN BONDS

A hydrogen bond is the attraction for a hydrogen atom by a highly electronegative element. The elements generally involved are fluorine, chlorine, oxygen, and nitrogen. Hydrogen bonds are the strongest of the intermolecular forces.

DIPOLE INTERACTIONS

Dipole interactions are the attractions of one dipole for another. A dipole is created when an electron pair in a covalent bond is shared unequally. The result is a bond in which the more highly electronegative element is slightly negative and the less electronegative element is slightly positive. The positive end of a dipole in one compound will be attracted to the negative end of another dipole in a separate compound. This attraction is considered a weak intermolecular force.

DISPERSION FORCES

Dispersion forces are the weakest of all intermolecular forces. Sometimes moving electrons within an element or compound concentrate themselves on one side of an atom. This causes a momentary dipole, which would be attracted to another momentary dipole in an adjoining element or compound. This attraction is called a *dispersion force*, and it is usually found in nonpolar covalent compounds.

Molar Relationships

One of the most important concepts in chemistry is the mole. A mole is the amount of a substance that contains 6.02×10^{23} representative particles of that substance. This is not unlike the word *dozen*, which is used to represent the number twelve. The mass of one mole of a substance is called the *atomic mass* and can be found on the periodic table. Depending on the desired unit, answers can be converted from one to another.

Through use of the atomic masses from the periodic table, it is possible to calculate the molar mass, or the mass of a mole of a compound.

Stoichiometry

The part of chemistry that deals with the quantities and the numeric relationships between compounds in a chemical reaction is called *stoichiometry*. For a chemical equation to be balanced, numbers called *coefficients* are placed in front of each compound. These numbers are used in a ratio to compare how much of one substance is needed to react with another in a certain reaction. The process is similar to comparing ingredients in a recipe.

$$2C_2H_6 + 7O_2 \rightarrow 4CO_2 + 6H_2O$$

Using this reaction, determine the number of moles of oxygen that will react with four moles of ethane (C_2H_6). Through use of a process called *dimensional analysis*, it is possible to convert from ethane to oxygen using a mole-to-mole ratio.

$$\frac{4 \text{ mol } C_2H_6}{} \left| \frac{7 \text{ mol } O_2}{2 \text{ mol } C_2H_6} \right. = 14 \text{ mol } O_2$$

The ratio of oxygen to ethane is seven to two. By multiplying the given amount of four moles of ethane by the ratio, one can determine the amount of oxygen needed to react. This method of multiplication can be used on a larger scale to convert from one unit to a variety of others.

Reaction Rates and Equilibrium

Not all chemical reactions proceed to completion; some simply slow down, with leftover amounts of reactant still present. These types of reactions are said to be *at equilibrium*. At this point, reactants are forming products at the same rate that products are forming reactants. The reaction is said to be *reversible*.

Through manipulation of the concentrations of the reactants or products, desired shifts in equilibrium can be achieved. A car battery is a good example. The battery produces electricity, but when charging, the opposite is true. With the addition of product (electricity), more reactant (a charged battery) is formed.

The rate of a reaction can be manipulated as well. There are four ways to increase the reaction rate: increase the temperature, increase the surface area, increase the concentrations of reactants, or add a catalyst.

INCREASING THE TEMPERATURE

Increasing the temperature causes the particles to have a greater kinetic energy, thereby enabling them to move faster and have a greater chance of contact. The contact is when chemical reactions occur.

INCREASING THE SURFACE AREA

Increasing the surface area gives particles more opportunity to come into contact with one another. Wood is an excellent example. Taking a log and cutting it into shavings or sawdust increases the rate of its reaction with the surrounding oxygen. Therefore the wood ignites and burns faster.

CONCENTRATIONS

Concentrating can be measured in several ways. One way is the weight or mass per volume unit, which is the amount of solute per volume of solution. This method is most often used when describing a solid that is being diluted by a liquid. Concentration can also be measured by volume per unit volume and is used when one liquid is diluted with another liquid. Concentration can be also be represented by a percentage and can be used with either liquids or solid chemicals. Another way to express concentration is by molarity of the solution or the gram-molecular mass of a compound per liter of solution. Finally, concentration can be expressed as osmolarity or the number of osmoles of solute per liter of solution. When the concentration is increased, the rate of the reaction is accelerated. Conversely when the concentration is decreased, the rate of the reaction is reduced.

> **HESI Hint** • Concentrations have a great deal to do with the rate of reaction. As is the case with males and females, increasing the numbers of reactants (persons) means that a greater number of collisions can take place.

CATALYSTS

A catalyst accelerates a reaction by reducing the activation energy, or the amount of energy necessary for a reaction to occur. The catalyst is not used up in the reaction and can be collected on reaction completion. Usually a car battery produces electricity. However, when the battery is being charged, the opposite is true. The battery then stores electricity in the form of chemical energy.

Oxidation and Reduction

Oxidation and reduction reactions are coupled together in a single term—*redox*. Redox reactions involve the transfer of electrons from one element to another. Oxidation is the loss of electrons, and

reduction is the gain of electrons. It is not possible to have one without the other.

To identify what has been oxidized and what has been reduced, the oxidation states of all elements in the compound must be determined. There is a series of steps to be followed to make that determination:

1. The oxidation number of any elemental atom is zero. This means that if an element is in its natural state, its number is zero. A good example is lead (Pb). Most elements in their standard states are single atoms, but a few exceptions exist. Those exceptions are H, Br, O, N, Cl, I, and F. These elements, when existing alone, are always in pairs. Oxygen would be O_2 and so forth.
2. The oxidation number of any simple ion is the charge of the ion. If in a reaction sodium were listed as an ion, Na^+, it would have an oxidation number of +1. If chlorine were listed as an ion, Cl^-, it would have an oxidation number of −1.
3. The oxidation number for oxygen in a compound is −2.
4. The oxidation number for hydrogen in a compound is +1.
5. The sum of the oxidation numbers equals the charge on the molecules or polyatomic ions.

Example: Assign oxidation numbers to all elements in the following reaction:

$$2C_2H_6 + 7O_2 \rightarrow 4CO_2 + 6H_2O$$

By using the rules listed earlier, we can use simple algebra to solve for the charges of those elements not discussed. Carbon will have to be determined. The first reactant is the compound C_2H_6. The coefficient of two has nothing to do with the oxidation state. The total charge on the compound is zero, as is determined using rule five. From rule four, hydrogen must have an oxidation state of +1. There are six of them, so the total charge of the hydrogen molecules is +6. Following is the algebra to solve for the oxidation state of carbon.

$$2x + 6(+1) = 0$$

Solving for x, carbon is found to have a charge of −3.

If the same method is used, the states of all the other elements can be determined. Oxygen in O_2 is zero (rule one). Carbon in CO_2 is +4, and oxygen is −2. Finally, hydrogen in water is +1, and oxygen is −2.

With this information it is possible to predict what is oxidized and what is reduced. Looking at the charges on either side of the equation, see what has changed. Carbon goes from a state of −3 to a state of +4. It has lost seven electrons and has therefore been oxidized. Oxygen's state has changed from 0 to −2. It has gained two electrons and has therefore been reduced.

Acids and Bases

Acids are those compounds acting as hydrogen-ion donors, and bases are those compounds acting as hydrogen ion acceptors.

Acids produce H_3O^+ in aqueous solutions, they taste sour or tart, most of their formulas begin with H, they release H_2 (g) when reacting with active metals, they conduct an electrical current, and they have a pH value less than 7. Bases produce OH^- in aqueous solutions, they taste bitter, they feel slippery, they conduct electricity, their formulas often contain OH^- in their names, and their pH is greater than 7. Figure 6-4 presents some examples of acids and bases on the pH range.

> **HESI Hint** • By manipulation of the quantity of acid and/or base in a solution, the pH can be altered. The process of neutralization occurs when an acid and a base react to produce a salt and water. Generally, this results in a neutral pH or a pH close to 7.

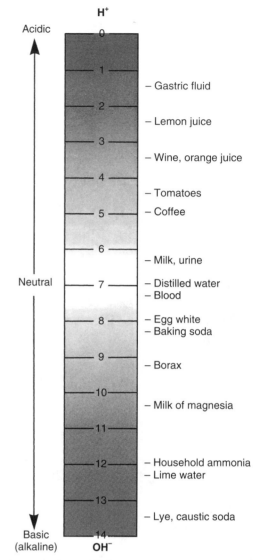

FIGURE 6-4 The pH range. (From Thibodeau GA, Patton KT: *Anatomy and physiology*, ed 5, St Louis, 2003, Mosby.)

Sample Chemistry Questions

1. What characterizes a chemical reaction as combustion?
    A. Formation of CO_2
    B. Addition of H_2
    C. Addition of O_2
    D. Formation of H_2O
2. What is the charge on potassium in the compound KCl?
    A. −1
    B. +1
    C. −2
    D. +2

3. How many electrons does an oxygen ion have?
   A. –2
   B. 8
   C. 10
   D. 2
4. How many neutrons does an atom of carbon-14 contain?
   A. 6
   B. 8
   C. 7
   D. 4
5. What is the strongest type of chemical bond?
   A. Covalent bond
   B. Hydrogen bond
   C. Ionic bond
   D. Dipole interaction
6. What is the mass of one mole of carbon dioxide?
   A. 44 g/mol
   B. 28 g/mol
   C. 56 g/mol
   D. 16 g/mol
7. How many molecules are present in two moles of O_2?
   A. 6.02×1023
   B. 1.204×1024
   C. 1.204×1021
   D. 6.02×10^{21}
8. Using the following equation, how many moles of CO_2 will be produced from the reaction of three moles of acetylene with excess oxygen?
$$2C_2H_2 + 5O_2 \rightarrow 4CO_2 + 2H_2O$$
   A. Two moles
   B. Four moles
   C. Six moles
   D. Eight moles
9. What would be the oxidation state of the sulfur atom in sulfuric acid, H_2SO_4?
   A. +4
   B. +5
   C. +6
   D. +8

Answers to Sample Chemistry Questions

1. C—*Combustion* is defined as the reaction of any compound or element with oxygen. Formation of CO_2 and formation of H_2O would be good choices if it was known that the reaction was a hydrocarbon producing CO_2 and H_2O.
2. B—Potassium (K) is in group IA and therefore has a +1 charge.
3. C—Oxygen has the atomic number 8. This means that it has eight protons. From its location on the periodic table, oxygen as an ion has a –2 charge. Therefore, the ion has two more electrons than protons. The oxygen ion must have 10 total electrons.
4. B—Because carbon has the atomic number 6, it has six protons. Given in the question is the mass number of carbon as well. The mass number is the sum of the protons and neutrons. So, by taking the difference of the mass number (14) and the atomic

number (6), one can determine the number of neutrons.

5. A—Covalent bond. The order of strength from strongest to weakest is covalent bond, ionic bond, hydrogen bond, dipole interaction, then, finally, dispersion forces.

6. A—The formula of carbon dioxide is CO_2. To calculate the molar mass, add the mass of one mole of carbon to the mass of two moles of oxygen.

7. B—1.204×10^{24} molecules. Because one mole of any substance is 6.02×10^{23} molecules, two moles would be twice that amount.

8. C—Determined by multiplying the given three moles of acetylene by the ratio, which in this case is four to two.

9. C—Hydrogen has a charge of $+1$, as stated in rule four, and oxygen has a charge of -2, as stated in rule three.

ANATOMY AND PHYSIOLOGY

7

Every student in the health professions should know the basics of anatomy and physiology. From cells and tissues to organs and systems, the human body is the most complex organism on earth. It is important that members of the health professions who take care of clients know how the human body works as a whole and what role specific parts of the body play in an individual's health and well-being.

A one-year course in anatomy and physiology should be taken before the student prepares for the anatomy examination. Take the time to read about anatomy and physiology at every opportunity. This preparation guide will go through each of the major body systems and point out the most important aspects of facts that should be learned.

General Terminology

Students of anatomy and physiology should learn some standard terms for body directions and subdivisions of the body. These will provide a basic introduction to the study of the body and also point out the need for the use of correct terminology.

The body planes are imaginary lines used for reference; they include the median plane, the coronal plane, and the transverse plane. A section is a real or imaginary cut made along a plane. A cut along the median plane is a sagittal section. A cut along the coronal plane is a frontal section, and a cut through the transverse plane is a cross-section. When describing the body, visualize the anatomical position. The body is erect, the feet are slightly apart, the head is held high, and the palms of the hands are facing forward.

Important terms of direction to review include *superior* (above), *inferior* (below), *anterior* (facing forward), *posterior* (toward the back), *medial* (toward the midline), and *lateral* (away from the midline or toward the sides). *Proximal* and *distal* are terms of direction usually used in reference to limbs. *Proximal* means closer to the point of attachment, and *distal* refers to further away from the point of attachment. Figure 7-1 depicts the directional terms.

Major body cavities are divided into the dorsal cavity (includes the cranial and spinal cavities) and the ventral cavity (includes the orbits and the nasal, oral, thoracic, and abdominopelvic cavities).

Additional useful terminology is defined later in this chapter.

Histology

Histology is the study of tissues. A tissue is a group of cells that act together to perform specific functions. The four fundamental tissues are epithelial, connective, muscle, and nerve tissues. Epithelial cells cover, line, and protect the body and its internal organs. Connective tissue is the framework of the body, providing support and structure for the organs. Nerve tissue is composed of neurons and connective tissue cells that are referred to as *neuroglia*. Muscle tissues have the ability to contract or shorten. Muscle tissue is classified as voluntary muscle (skeletal muscles)

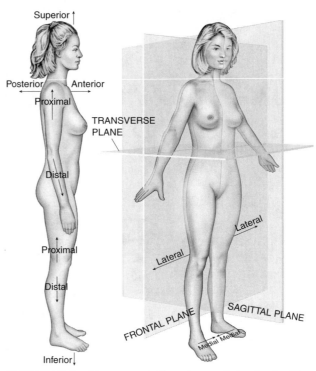

FIGURE 7-1 Planes and directions of the body. (From Thibodeau GA, Patton KT: *Anatomy and physiology*, ed 6, St Louis, 2007, Mosby.)

or involuntary muscle (smooth muscle and cardiac muscle tissue).

The major parts of the cell should be reviewed. The cell is the basic unit of life and the building block of tissues and organs. Within the cell each organelle has a specific function. The nucleus, which contains deoxyribonucleic acid (DNA), and ribosomes are especially important in the synthesis of proteins. Proteins include the enzymes that regulate all chemical reactions within the body.

Mitosis and Meiosis

Mitosis is necessary for growth and repair. In this process the DNA is duplicated and distributed evenly to two daughter cells. Meiosis is the special cell division that takes place in the gonads, that is, the ovaries and testes. In the process of meiosis the chromosome number is reduced from 46 to 23, so when the egg and the sperm unite in fertilization the zygote will have the correct number of chromosomes.

Membranes, Glands, and Cartilage

Mucous, serous, synovial, and cutaneous are the principal kinds of membranes and are composed mainly of epithelial tissue. Types of glands include sudoriferous, sebaceous, and ceruminous. Cartilage is replaced by bone in embryonic development and is found mainly in the joints, the thorax, and various rigid tubes.

Skin

The skin is the largest organ of the body. The skin consists of two layers: the epidermis (the outermost protective layer of dead keratinized epithelial cells) and the dermis (the underlying layer of connective tissue with blood vessels, nerve endings, and the associated skin structures). The dermis rests on the subcutaneous tissue that connects the skin to the superficial muscles.

The layers of the epidermis, from outer layer to inner layer, are the stratum corneum, the stratum lucidum, the stratum granulosum, and the innermost stratum germinativum, where mitosis occurs. Epidermal cells contain the protein pigment called *melanin*, which protects against radiation from the sun.

The inner layer of the skin is the dermis, composed of fibrous connective tissue with blood vessels, sensory nerve endings, hair follicles, and glands. There are two types of sweat glands. The most widely distributed sweat glands regulate body temperature by releasing a watery secretion that evaporates from the surface of the skin. This type of sweat gland is known as *eccrine*. The other sweat glands, mainly in the armpits and groin area, display apocrine secretion. This secretion contains bits of cytoplasm from the secreting cells. This cell debris attracts bacteria, and the presence of the bacteria on the skin results in body odor. The sebaceous glands release an oily secretion (sebum) through the hair follicles that lubricates the skin and prevents drying. Oil is produced by holocrine secretion, in which whole cells of the gland are part of the secretion. These glands are susceptible to becoming clogged and attracting bacteria, particularly during adolescence.

The appendages of the skin include hair and nails. Both are composed of a strong protein called *keratin*.

Hair, nails, and skin may show changes in disease that may be used in the diagnosis of clinical conditions. For example, skin cancer is a clinical condition that is associated with the skin.

Skeletal System

The body framework consists of bone, cartilage, and ligaments, plus the joints between the bones. Functions of the skeletal system include support, permission of movement, blood cell formation (hemopoiesis), protection of internal organs, detoxification (removal of poisons), provision for muscle attachment, and mineral storage (particularly calcium and phosphorus).

Individual bones are classified by shape. There are long bones, short bones, flat bones, irregular bones, and sesamoid bones, such as the patella. A typical long bone has an irregular epiphysis at each end, composed mainly of spongy (cancellous) bone, and a shaft or diaphysis, composed mainly of compact bone. The cells that form compact bone are called *osteoblasts;* when they become fixed in the dense bone matrix, they stop dividing but continue to maintain bone tissue as osteocytes.

The axial skeleton (Figure 7-2) consists of the 28 bones of the skull. These are separated into the 14 facial bones and the 14 bones of the cranium. The facial bones are two nasal bones, two maxillary bones, two zygomatic bones, one mandible (the only moveable bone of the skull), two palatine bones, one vomer, two lacrimal bones, and two inferior nasal conchae. The bones of the cranium are the single occipital, frontal, ethmoid, and sphenoid and the paired parietal, temporal, and ossicles of the ear (malleus, incus, and stapes).

The axial skeleton also has 33 bones of the vertebral column, as depicted in Figure 7-3. There are seven cervical vertebrae, 12 thoracic vertebrae, five lumbar vertebrae, five sacral vertebrae (fused to form the sacrum), and the coccygeal vertebrae (known as the *tailbone*). The final portion of the axial skeleton consists of the bones of the thorax, the sternum, and the 12 pairs of ribs.

The appendicular skeleton (see Figure 7-2) includes the girdles and the limbs. The upper portion consists of the pectoral or shoulder girdle, the clavicle and scapula, and the upper extremity. The bones of the arm are the humerus, the radius and ulna, the carpals (wrist bones), the metacarpals

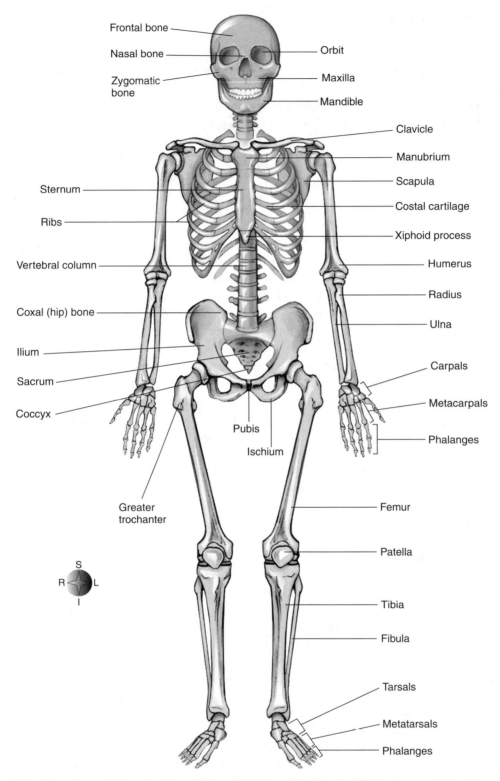

FIGURE 7-2 **Anterior view of the skeleton.** (From Thibodeau GA, Patton KT: *Anatomy and physiology,* ed 6, St Louis, 2007, Mosby.)

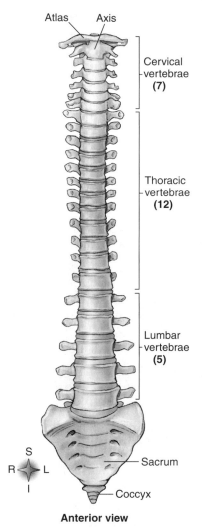

Atlas   Axis

Cervical
vertebrae
(7)

Thoracic
vertebrae
(12)

Lumbar
vertebrae
(5)

S
R ✦ L
I

Sacrum

Coccyx

Anterior view

FIGURE 7-3 Anterior view of the vertebral column.
(From Thibodeau GA, Patton KT: *Anatomy and physiology*, ed 6,
St Louis, 2007, Mosby.)

myosin filaments within the muscle cell or fiber. Each muscle cell consists of myofibrils, which in turn are made up of still smaller units called *sarcomeres*. In order for a muscle cell to contract, calcium and adenosine triphosphate (ATP) must be present. Nervous stimulation from motor neurons causes the release of calcium ions from the sarcoplasmic reticulum. Calcium ions attach to inhibitory proteins on the actin filaments within the cell, moving them aside so that cross-bridges can form between actin and myosin filaments. Using energy supplied by ATP, the filaments slide together to produce contraction.

The skeletal muscles, which make up the muscular system, are also called *voluntary muscles* because they are under conscious control. Skeletal muscles must work in pairs: the muscle that executes a given movement is the prime mover, whereas the muscle that produces the opposite movement is the antagonist. Other muscles known as *synergists* may work in cooperation with the prime mover.

Muscles can be classified according to the movements they elicit. There are flexors and extensors. Flexors reduce the angle at the joint, whereas extensors increase the angle. Abductors draw a limb away from the midline, and adductors return the limb back toward the body.

> **HESI Hint** • Starting at the head and moving to the feet, name the major contour muscles of the body. Review how muscles are named—some for their function, others for their location or for the numbers of points of origin.

(bones of the hand), and the phalanges (bones of the fingers). The lower portion of the appendicular skeleton is made up of the pelvic girdle or *os coxae*. Each of the os coxae consists of a fused ilium, ischium, and pubis. Bones of the lower extremity include the femur (thighbone), the tibia and fibula, the tarsals (ankle bones), the metatarsals (bones of the foot), and the phalanges.

Muscular System

Muscles produce movement by contracting in response to nervous stimulation. Muscle contraction results from the sliding together of actin and

Nervous System

The nervous system consists essentially of the brain, the spinal cord, and the nerves (Figure 7-4). This vital system enables us to perceive many of the changes that take place in our external and internal environments and to respond to those changes (seeing, hearing, tasting, smelling, and touching are examples of perception). It enables us to think, reason, remember, and carry out other abstract activities. It makes possible body movements by skeletal muscles, by supplying them with nerve impulses that cause contraction. It works closely with the endocrine glands,

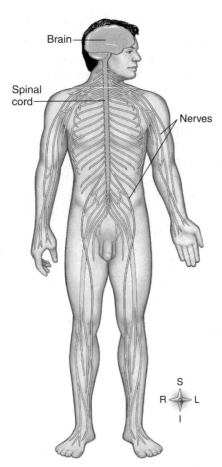

FIGURE 7-4 **Major anatomic features of the nervous system include the brain, the spinal cord, and the individual nerves. The central nervous system (CNS) consists of the brain and spinal cord. The peripheral nervous system (PNS) includes all of the nerves and their branches.** (From Thibodeau GA, Patton KT: *Anatomy and physiology*, ed 6, St Louis, 2007, Mosby.)

correlating and integrating body functions such as digestion and reproduction.

All actions of the nervous system depend on the transmission of nerve impulses over neurons, or nerve cells, the functional units of the nervous system. The main parts of a neuron are the cell body, axon, and dendrites. Dendrites transmit the impulse toward the cell body, and axons transmit the impulse away from the cell body.

The nervous system may be divided structurally into a central nervous system (CNS) and a peripheral nervous system (PNS) (see Figure 7-4). The PNS consists of all the nerves that transmit information to and from the CNS. Sensory (afferent) neurons transmit nerve impulses toward the CNS. Motor (efferent) neurons transmit nerve impulses away

from the CNS, toward the effector organs such as muscles, glands, and digestive organs.

The major parts of the brain are the cerebrum (associated with movement and sensory input), the cerebellum (responsible for muscular coordination), and the medulla oblongata (controls many vital functions such as respiration and heart rate).

The spinal cord is approximately 18 inches long and extends from the base of the skull (foramen magnum) to the first or second lumbar vertebra (L1 or L2). Thirty-one pairs of spinal nerves exit the spinal cord. Simple (spinal) reflexes are those in which nerve impulses travel through the spinal cord only and do not reach the brain.

> **HESI Hint** • Most reflex pathways involve impulses traveling to and from the brain in ascending and descending tracts of the spinal cord. Sensory impulses enter the dorsal horns of the spinal cord, and motor impulses leave through the ventral horns of the spinal cord.

Endocrine System

The endocrine system assists the nervous system in homeostasis and plays important roles in growth and sexual maturation. These two systems meet at the hypothalamus and pituitary gland. The hypothalamus governs the pituitary and is in turn controlled by the feedback of hormones in the blood. The nervous and endocrine systems coordinate and control the body, but the endocrine system has more long-lasting and widespread effects.

Hormones are chemical messengers that control the growth, differentiation, and metabolism of specific target cells. There are two major groups of hormones. Steroid hormones enter the target cells and have a direct effect on the DNA of the nucleus. Most protein hormones remain at the cell surface and act through a second messenger, usually a substance called *adenosine mono phosphate* (AMP). Most hormones affect cell activity by altering the rate of protein synthesis.

The endocrine glands, although widely distributed, are grouped together as a system because the main function of each gland is the production of hormones. Other organs, such as the stomach, small intestine, and kidneys, produce hormones as well.

The pituitary gland is nicknamed the *master gland*. It is attached to the hypothalamus by a stalk called the *infundibulum*. The pituitary gland has two major portions: the anterior lobe (adenohypophysis) and the posterior lobe (neurohypophysis). Hormones of the adenohypophysis are called *tropic hormones* because they act mainly on other endocrine glands. They include:

- Somatotropin (STH) or growth hormone (GH)
- Adrenocorticotropic hormone (ACTH)
- Thyroid-stimulating hormone (TSH)
- Follicle-stimulating hormone (FSH)
- Luteinizing hormone (LH)

Hormones released from the posterior lobe of the pituitary include oxytocin (the labor hormone) and antidiuretic hormone (ADH).

Other important endocrine glands include the thyroid, parathyroids, adrenals, pancreas, and gonads (the ovaries and testes).

Circulatory System

Whole blood consists of approximately 55% plasma and 45% formed elements: erythrocytes (red blood cells), leukocytes (white blood cells), and platelets. All of the formed elements are produced from stem cells in red bone marrow. Erythrocytes are modified for transport of oxygen. Most of this oxygen is bound to the pigmented protein hemoglobin. The five types of leukocytes can be distinguished on the basis of size, appearance of the nucleus, staining properties, and presence or absence of visible cytoplasmic granules. White blood cells are active in phagocytosis (neutrophils and monocytes) and antibody formation (lymphocytes). Platelets are active in the process of blood clotting.

Blood serves to transport oxygen and nutrients to body cells and to carry away carbon dioxide and metabolic wastes. Plasma contains approximately 10% proteins, ions, nutrients, waste products, and hormones, which are dissolved or suspended in water.

The heart is a double pump that sends blood to the lungs for oxygenation through the pulmonary circuit and to the remainder of the body through the systemic circuit.

Blood is received by the atria and is pumped into circulation by the ventricles. Valves between the atria and ventricles include the tricuspid on the right side of the heart and the bicuspid on the left. Semilunar valves are found at the entrances of the pulmonary trunk and the aorta. Blood is supplied to the heart muscle (the myocardium) by the coronary arteries. Blood drains from the myocardium directly into the right atrium through the coronary sinus.

The heart has an intrinsic beat initiated by the sinoatrial node and transmitted along a conduction system through the myocardium. This wave of electrical activity is what is measured on an electrocardiogram (ECG). The cardiac cycle is the period from the end of one ventricular contraction to the end of the next ventricular contraction. The contraction phase of the cycles is systole; the relaxation phase is diastole.

The vascular system includes arteries that carry blood away from the heart, veins that carry blood toward the heart, and the microscopic vessels (the capillaries) through which exchanges take place between the blood and the cells of the body. The systemic arteries begin with the aorta, which sends branches to all parts of the body. As arteries get farther away from the heart, they become thinner and thinner. The smallest arteries are called *arterioles*. The veins parallel the arteries and usually have the same names. The superior and inferior venae cavae are the large veins that empty into the right atrium of the heart.

The walls of the arteries are thick and elastic, and they carry blood under high pressure. Vasoconstriction and vasodilation result from contraction and relaxation of smooth muscle in the arterial walls. These changes influence blood pressure and blood distribution to the tissues. The walls of the veins are thinner and less elastic than those of the arteries, and they carry blood under lower pressure.

> **HESI Hint** • Mechanisms that help to draw venous blood back to the heart include pressure of the skeletal muscles on the veins, expansion of the chest in breathing, and valves in the veins of the legs that keep blood moving in a forward direction.

> **HESI Hint** • Review the major arteries and veins of the body.

Respiratory System

Components of the respiratory system include the nose, pharynx, larynx, trachea, bronchi, lungs with their alveoli, diaphragm, and muscles surrounding the ribs. Respiration is controlled by the respiratory control center in the medulla of the brain.

The respiratory system supplies oxygen to the body and eliminates carbon dioxide. *External respiration* refers to the exchange of gases between the atmosphere and the blood through the alveoli. *Internal respiration* refers to the exchange of gases between the blood and the body cells. The passageways between the nasal cavities and the alveoli conduct gases to and from the lungs. The upper passageways also serve to warm, filter, and moisten incoming air. These upper respiratory tubules are lined with cilia that help to trap debris and keep foreign substances from entering the lungs.

Inhalation requires the contraction of the diaphragm to enlarge the chest cavity and draw air into the lungs. Exhalation is a passive process during which the lungs recoil as the respiratory muscles relax and the thorax decreases in size.

Most of the oxygen carried in the blood is bound to hemoglobin in red blood cells. Oxygen is released from hemoglobin as the concentration of oxygen drops in the tissues. Some carbon dioxide is carried in solution or bound to blood proteins, but most is converted to bicarbonate ion by carbonic anhydrase within red blood cells. Because this reaction also releases hydrogen ions, carbon dioxide is a regulator of blood pH.

> **HESI Hint**
> • List the respiratory organs.
> • Trace the pathways of oxygen and carbon dioxide.
> • Describe the process of gas exchange.

Digestive System

The alimentary canal or digestive tube consists of the mouth, pharynx, esophagus, stomach, small intestine, large intestine, rectum, and anus. The accessory organs of digestion include the liver, pancreas, and gallbladder.

Food is ingested into the mouth, where it is mechanically broken down by the teeth and tongue in the process of mastication (chewing). Saliva, produced by the three pairs of salivary glands, lubricates and dilutes the chewed food. Saliva contains an enzyme called *amylase* that starts the digestion of complex carbohydrates. A ball of food called a *bolus* is formed. Constrictive muscles of the pharynx force the food into the upper portion of the esophagus, and the food is swallowed. The esophagus is a narrow tube leading from the pharynx to the stomach. The digestive tract has four main layers, from inner to outer: the mucous membrane, the submucous layer, the muscular layer, and the serous layer.

Food enters the stomach, where gastric glands secrete hydrochloric acid that breaks down foods. The stomach muscle churns and mixes the bolus of food, turning the mass into a soupy substance called *chyme*. The stomach also stores food and regulates the movement of food into the small intestine.

Almost all digestion and absorption of food occurs in the small intestine. Here, food is acted on by various enzymes from the small intestine and pancreas and by bile from the liver. The pancreas also contributes water to dilute the chyme and bicarbonate ions to neutralize the acid from the stomach. The small intestine consists of three major regions: the duodenum, the jejunum, and the ileum. Nutrients are absorbed through the walls of the small intestine. The amino acids and simple sugars derived from proteins and

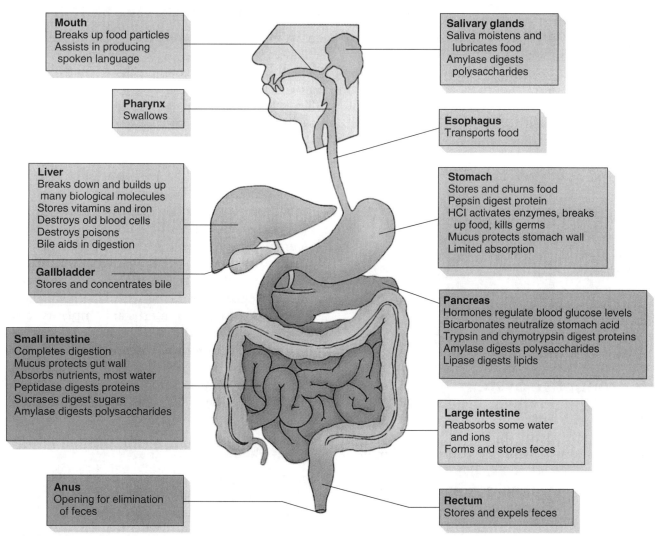

Mouth
Breaks up food particles
Assists in producing
  spoken language

Salivary glands
Saliva moistens and
  lubricates food
Amylase digests
  polysaccharides

Pharynx
Swallows

Esophagus
Transports food

Liver
Breaks down and builds up
  many biological molecules
Stores vitamins and iron
Destroys old blood cells
Destroys poisons
Bile aids in digestion

Gallbladder
Stores and concentrates bile

Stomach
Stores and churns food
Pepsin digest protein
HCl activates enzymes, breaks
  up food, kills germs
Mucus protects stomach wall
Limited absorption

Pancreas
Hormones regulate blood glucose levels
Bicarbonates neutralize stomach acid
Trypsin and chymotrypsin digest proteins
Amylase digests polysaccharides
Lipase digests lipids

Small intestine
Completes digestion
Mucus protects gut wall
Absorbs nutrients, most water
Peptidase digests proteins
Sucrases digest sugars
Amylase digests polysaccharides

Large intestine
Reabsorbs some water
  and ions
Forms and stores feces

Anus
Opening for elimination
  of feces

Rectum
Stores and expels feces

FIGURE 7-5   Summary of the vital and nonvital roles of digestion. (From Thibodeau GA, Patton KT: *Anatomy and physiology,* ed 6, St Louis, 2007, Mosby.)

carbohydrates are absorbed directly into the blood. Most of the fats are absorbed into the lymph by the lacteals, which eventually are added to the bloodstream. All nutrients then enter the hepatic portal vein to be routed to the liver for decontamination. Small fingerlike projections called *villi* greatly increase the surface area of the intestinal wall.

The large intestine reabsorbs water and stores and eliminates undigested food. Here also are abundant bacteria, the intestinal flora. The large intestine is arranged into five portions: the ascending colon, the transverse colon, the descending colon, the sigmoid colon, and the rectum. The opening for defecation (expelling of stool) is the anus.

The roles of the various organs are summarized in Figure 7-5.

Urinary System

The urinary system consists of two kidneys, two ureters, a urinary bladder, and the urethra. The kidneys filter the blood. The ureters are tubes that transport urine to the urinary bladder, where urine is stored before urination through the urethra to the outside.

The functional units of the kidney are the nephrons. These small coiled tubes filter waste material out of blood brought to the kidney by the renal artery. The actual filtration process occurs through the glomerulus in Bowman's capsule of the nephron. Filtration of the blood occurs through the glomerulus under the force of blood pressure. As the glomerular filtrate passes through the nephron, components needed by the body, such as water, glucose, and ions, leave the nephron by diffusion and reenter the blood. Water is reabsorbed at the tubules of the nephron. The final product produced by the millions of nephrons per kidney is urine.

> **HESI Hint**
> • Describe the functions of the components of the urinary system: the kidneys, ureters, urinary bladder, and urethra. (Note that the male urethra is also part of the reproductive system.)
> • Review the ultrastructure of the nephron and the process of urine formation.

Reproductive System

The male and female sex organs (the testes and ovaries) have two functions: production of gametes (sex cells) and production of hormones. These activities are under the control of tropic hormones from the pituitary gland. Reproductive activity is cyclic in women but continuous in men. The gametes are formed by meiosis.

MALE REPRODUCTIVE SYSTEM

In men, spermatozoa develop within the seminiferous tubules of each testis. The interstitial cells between the seminiferous tubules produce testosterone. This male hormone influences sperm cell development and also produces the male secondary sex characteristics such as body hair and deep voice. Once produced, the sperm are stored in the epididymis of each testis. During ejaculation the pathway for the sperm includes the vas deferens, ejaculatory duct, and urethra. Along the pathway are glands that produce the transport medium or semen. These include the seminal vesicles, prostate gland, and bulbourethral (Cowper's) glands. Testicular activity is under the control of two anterior pituitary hormones. FSH stimulates sperm production. Interstitial cell-stimulating hormone (ICSH) or LH stimulates the interstitial cells to produce testosterone.

FEMALE REPRODUCTIVE SYSTEM

In women, each month, under the influence of FSH, several eggs ripen within the ovarian follicles in the ovary. The estrogen produced by the follicle initiates the preparation of the endometrium of the uterus for pregnancy. At approximately day 14 of the cycle, LH is released from the pituitary, which stimulates ovulation and the conversion of the follicle to the corpus luteum. The corpus luteum secretes the hormone progesterone, which further stimulates development of the endometrium. If fertilization occurs, the corpus luteum remains functional. If fertilization does not occur, the corpus luteum degenerates and menstruation begins.

After ovulation the egg is swept into the oviduct or fallopian tube. If fertilization occurs, it occurs while the egg is in the oviduct. The fertilized egg or zygote travels to the uterus and implants itself within the endometrium. In the uterus the developing embryo is nourished by the placenta, which is formed by maternal and embryonic tissues. During pregnancy, hormones from the placenta maintain the endometrium and prepare the breasts for milk production.

> **HESI Hint**
> • List the organs of the male reproductive system.
> • List the organs of the female reproductive system
> • Describe the events of the menstrual cycle.

Helpful Terminology

Abdominopelvic: Cavity composed of the abdomen and the pelvis.
Absorption: Movement of nutrients from the digestive tube into the bloodstream.
Actin: Protein making up the I band of the sarcomere.
Amino Acid: The building block of proteins.
Antibody: Special proteins that protect the body from foreign substances.
ATP: Abbreviation for adenosine triphosphate, which is the energy of the cell.
Atria: Upper chambers of the heart.
Bile: Product of the liver that emulsifies fat.
Cartilage: Tissue made of cells and fibers that connect and support.
Ceruminous Gland: Gland of the ear that produces earwax.

Chromosomes: Bodies within the nucleus made of DNA and proteins called *histones*.

Cilia: Small hairlike projections on some cells.

CNS: Abbreviation for central nervous system, which is made up of the brain and spinal cord.

Coronal Plane: Imaginary line passing through the body from head to feet that divides the body into front and back portions.

Cranial Cavity: Body cavity containing the brain.

Diaphragm: Dome-shaped breathing muscle that separates the thoracic and abdominal cavities.

Diffusion: Movement of materials from high concentration to lower concentration.

Digestion: The mechanical and chemical breakdown of food.

Dorsal Horn: Crescent-shaped projection of gray matter within the spinal cord where sensory neurons enter the spinal cord.

ECG: Abbreviation for electrocardiogram, which is a record of the electrical activity of the heart.

Embryo: Prenatal development time between the zygote and the fetus.

Endometrium: Inner lining of the uterus.

Enzymes: Functional proteins; their names usually end in *ase*.

Foramen Magnum: A passage in the skull bone through which the spinal cord enters the spinal column.

Formed Elements: The blood cells.

Glucose: A simple sugar found in certain foods, especially fruits.

Homeostasis: The physiologic steady state that is naturally maintained within the body.

Hypothalamus: Portion of the brain that regulates body temperature, sleep, and appetite.

Ingest: To eat food and drink.

Joints: Articulations between adjoining bones.

Keratin: A tough, fibrous, insoluble protein forming the primary component of skin, hair, nails, and tooth enamel.

Keratinized Epithelium: The dead cells of the epidermis.

Lacteal Vessel: Found within the villi of intestinal wall, where fat nutrients are absorbed.

Ligaments: Tissue connecting bone to bone.

Median Plane: An imaginary line dividing the body or body part into right and left portions.

Mediastinum: Space within the thoracic cavity that houses all the organs of the chest except the lungs.

Metabolism: The sum total of uses of ATP in the body.

Mucous Membrane: Thin sheets of tissue cells that line body openings or canals that open to the outside of the body.

Myosin: A protein that makes up nearly half of the proteins in muscle cells.

Nucleus: The control center of the cell.

Oral Cavity: The mouth; also known as the *buccal cavity*.

Orbits: Cavities containing the eyes.

Organelle: A structurally discrete component of a cell that performs a specific function.

pH: Measurement associated with acids and bases.

Phagocytosis: Engulfing of materials by certain cells of the body.

Plasma: The liquid portion of blood.

Pulmonary Circulation: Blood flow through a network of vessels between the heart and the lungs for the oxygenation of blood and the removal of carbon dioxide.

Ribosome: The organelle of the cell where protein synthesis takes place.

Sagittal: An imaginary line running from front to back that divides the body into right and left portions.

Sarcoplasmic Reticulum: Organelle of the muscle fiber that stores calcium.

Sebaceous Glands: Oil glands of the skin.

Serous Membranes: Thin sheets of tissue that line body cavities not having exits to the outside.

Spinal Column: The backbone that protects the spinal cord, which runs inside of it.

Subcutaneous Tissue: Layer of tissue under the dermis that contains adipose tissue.

Sudoriferous Glands: Sweat glands.

Synovial Membranes: Loose, connective tissue that lines the joint cavity.

Systemic Circulation: The general blood circulation of the body, not including the lungs.

Thoracic Cavity: The chest cavity.

Transverse Plane: An imaginary line dividing the body or body parts into top and bottom portions.

Vasoconstriction: A narrowing of the diameter of a blood vessel.

Vasodilation: A widening of the diameter of a blood vessel.

Ventral Horns: The anterior columns of the gray matter of the spinal cord.

Ventricles: Lower chambers of the heart.

Zygote: The fertilized egg, from the time it is fertilized until it is implanted in the uterus.

Sample Anatomy and Physiology Questions

1. Using anatomic directions, describe the location of the ankle in relation to the knee.
   A. Anterior
   B. Posterior
   C. Proximal
   D. Distal

2. What is the serous membrane surrounding the heart called?
   A. Peritoneum
   B. Pleura
   C. Pericardium
   D. Pronator

3. What is the actively mitotic layer of the epidermis called?
   A. Stratum granulosum
   B. Stratum germinativum
   C. Stratum corium
   D. Stratum corneum

4. What is the total number of phalanges in the skeleton?
   A. 14
   B. 28
   C. 42
   D. 56

5. The flexor carpi ulnaris is located in what part of the body?
   A. Neck
   B. Wrist
   C. Hip
   D. Knee

6. What area of the brain controls muscle coordination and balance?
   A. Cerebellum
   B. Cerebrum
   C. Medulla
   D. Hypothalamus

7. What is the nickname for the pituitary gland, which produces tropic hormones?
   A. The slave driver
   B. The metabolism master
   C. The fight-or-flight hormone
   D. The master gland

8. Which of the following is not a type of white blood cell?
   A. Erythrocytes
   B. Neutrophils
   C. Lymphocytes
   D. Monocytes

9. What cellular structures trap bacteria and pollutants in the upper respiratory system?
   A. Flagella
   B. Microvilli
   C. Cilia
   D. Centrioles

10. What is the largest gland of the human body?
    A. Pancreas
    B. Spleen
    C. Gall bladder
    D. Liver
11. What structure acts as a storage area for urine?
    A. Kidney
    B. Ureter
    C. Urinary bladder
    D. Urethra
12. What portion of the uterus is under direct hormonal effect?
    A. Endometrium
    B. Myometrium
    C. Fundus
    D. Cervix

Answers to Sample Anatomy and Physiology Questions

1. D—The ankle is further away from the trunk of the body than is the knee. The term for this is distal.
2. C—Peri means "around"; cardio refers to the heart. The membrane around the heart would be the pericardium.
3. B—Stratum germinativum. When a seed germinates, it grows; growth is achieved through mitosis.
4. D—Each hand has 14 phalanges and each foot has 14 phalanges.
5. B—The muscle flexes the wrist toward the ulna.
6. A—The cerebellum controls muscle coordination and balance.
7. D—Tropic hormones affect other endocrine glands, so the pituitary is nicknamed the *master gland*.
8. A—Erythrocytes are red blood cells.
9. C—Cilia are present in the respiratory tract as well as in the fallopian tubes of the female.
10. D—The liver is the chemical factory and the largest gland of the body.
11. C—The walls of the urinary bladder are composed of transitional epithelia, which are able to expand.
12. A—Estrogen and progesterone both stimulate monthly proliferation of the endometrium.

RITE AID PHARMACY

With us, it's personal.

Store #07879
5455 RIDGE RD
PARMA, OH 44129
(440) 886-2148

Register #2 Transaction #279262
Cashier #78797822 11/09/10 2:07PM

1 Items

1 PASSPORT PHOTO   7.99 T

                Subtotal   7.99
                     Tax   .62
                   Total   8.61

*VISA *
   VISA   card * #XXXXXXXXXXXXX2432
   App # AUTO
   Ref # 00583C
   Card Present

                Tendered   8.61
             Cash Change   .00

T - Taxable

****

ENROLL TODAY in wellness+
and Save Everyday!!

PHYSICS

8

Members of the health professions, particularly those involved in imaging science such as radiographers, use the fundamental principles of physics on a daily basis as they relate to imaging science, radiation safety, radiation limits, client and health professional shielding, client positioning, and a host of other requirements related to their clients. Safety and high-quality image production are the goals of all who work within the imaging sciences as health professions. Therefore it is essential that students entering the health professions as radiographers understand the fundamental principles of physics related to heat, waves, and motion.

The purpose of this chapter is to review the fundamentals of physics related to linear motion, rotational motion, Newton's laws of motion, electrical fields, waves, kinetic energy, and potential energy. Mastery of these basic principles of physics is an integral step toward a career as a health professional in imaging science.

Average Speed

A study of the behavior of matter begins with understanding of the nature of motion. The most fundamental concept to comprehend is average speed. *Average speed* is defined as the distance an object travels divided by the time the object travels. This concept is represented mathematically by the following equation, where v_{av} = average speed, d = distance, and t = time.

$$\text{Average speed } (v_{av}) = \frac{\text{Distance}}{\text{Time}} = \frac{d}{t}$$

An important related concept is velocity. *Velocity* refers to speed in a specific direction. Speed is a scalar quantity and is expressed in units of magnitude. Velocity is a vector quantity and must be expressed in both units of magnitude (i.e., speed) and direction of the object of interest.

The average speed of an object is determined by averaging the initial speed and the final speed of the object. This concept is represented mathematically by the following equation, where v_f = final velocity and v_i = initial velocity.

$$v_{av} = \frac{v_f + v_i}{2}$$

Sample Problem

1. A car moves for 10 minutes and travels 5,280 meters. What is the average speed of the car?
   A. 528 m/sec
   B. 52.8 m/sec
   C. 8.8 m/sec
   D. 88 m/sec

Answer

1. C—Dividing the distance traveled by the car (5280 meters) by the new value for time traveled by the car (600 seconds) determines that the average speed of the care is 8.8 m/sec.

$$\text{Average speed } (v_{av}) = \frac{\text{Distance}}{\text{Time}}$$

$$\text{Average speed} = \frac{5280 \text{ m}}{600 \text{ sec}}$$

$$\text{Average speed} = 8.8 \text{ m/sec}$$

Average speed is the distance an object travels divided by the time the object travels. The answers must be expressed in m/sec; therefore the time of travel by the car must be converted from minutes to seconds before the average speed is determined.

$$\frac{x}{10 \text{ min}} = \frac{60 \text{sec}}{1 \text{ min}}$$

$$x = \frac{60 \text{ sec} \times 10 \text{ min}}{1 \text{ min}}$$

$$x = 600 \text{ sec}$$

Acceleration

Objects can have motions that are a little more complex than average speed. Often, objects change their speed over a period of time. This motion is called *acceleration* and is defined as the change in velocity over period of time. Acceleration is a vector quantity and is expressed in terms of magnitude and direction. This concept is represented mathematically by the following equation, where a = acceleration, v_f = final velocity, v_i = initial velocity, and Δt = the change in time.

$$\text{Acceleration} (a) = \frac{\Delta \text{ Velocity}}{\Delta \text{ Time}} = \frac{\Delta v}{\Delta t} = \frac{v_f - v_i}{\Delta t}$$

Sample Problem

2. A cart is set into motion. The cart has an initial speed of 15 m/sec and moves for 25 seconds. At the end of 25 seconds, the cart's speed is 40 m/sec. What is the magnitude of the cart's acceleration?
   A. 1.0 m/sec²
   B. 2.2 m/sec²
   C. 10.0 m/sec²
   D. 1.1 m/sec²

Answer

2. A—Acceleration is determined by dividing the change in the cart's velocity (25 m/sec) by the length of time the cart was in motion (25 seconds), indicating the cart is accelerating at 1.0 m/sec².

$$\text{Acceleration}(a) = \frac{v_f - v_i}{\Delta t}$$

$$a = \frac{40 \text{ m/sec} - 13 \text{ m/sec}}{24 \text{ sec}}$$

$$a = \frac{25 \text{ m/sec}}{25 \text{ sec}}$$

$$a = 1.0 \text{ m/sec}^2$$

It is possible to combine the basic mathematic expressions for speed, velocity, and acceleration to provide additional expressions that help explain the motion of an object. Familiarity with the following mathematical expressions may be helpful when solving more complex problems associated with the motion of objects.

$$v_f^2 = v_i^2 + 2ad$$

$$d = \tfrac{1}{2}at^2 + v_i t$$

$$v_f = v_i + at$$

Sample Problem

3. A ball is rolling down a hill with an initial speed of 6.0 m/sec. The ball accelerates at the rate of 1.5 m/sec² for 8.0 seconds. Determine the magnitude of the ball's displacement at the end of 8.0 seconds.
   A. 54.0 m
   B. 96.0 m
   C. 48.0 m
   D. 24.0 m

Answer

3. B—To determine the magnitude of the ball's displacement use the following equation:

$$d = \tfrac{1}{2}at^2 + v_i t$$

It is critical to square the time value in the first portion of the equation to accurately calculate the distance the ball traveled. Inserting the appropriate values into the equation indicates the ball traveled 96.0 meters in the 8-second time interval.

$$d = \tfrac{1}{2}at^2 + v_i t$$

$$d = \tfrac{1}{2}(1.5 \text{ m/sec}^2)(8.0 \text{ sec})^2 + (6.0 \text{ m/sec})(8.0 \text{ sec})$$

$$d = \tfrac{1}{2}(96 \text{ m}) + (48 \text{ m})$$

$$d = 96 \text{ m}$$

Projectile Motion

The acceleration of objects released above the surface of the earth is influenced by the force of gravity. Gravity, assuming no wind resistance, accelerates an object released above the earth's surface at a rate of 9.8 m/sec². For example, if a rock is released from rest and falls toward the earth, the speed of the rock will increase by 9.8 m/sec for every second the object falls. At the end of three seconds the object will have a speed of 29.4 m/sec and a velocity of 29.4 m/sec in the direction toward Earth's surface.

It is also possible for an object to display two types of motion simultaneously. This motion is generally called *projectile motion*. If a can is kicked from the edge of a cliff, the can will move horizontally at the same time it falls toward Earth. The horizontal motion is not an accelerated motion; therefore horizontal distance (d_x) is a function of velocity (v_x) and time (t) based on the following mathematic expression, where the x subscript is used to denote motion along the horizontal plane (x axis).

$$d_x = v_x t$$

The vertical motion is more complicated. Gravity is acting vertically, so the motion along the vertical plane (y axis) is constantly changing. The following mathematic expressions represent several methods of describing vertical motion, where v_f = final velocity, v_i = initial velocity, a = acceleration, d = distance, and t = time.

$$v_f^2 = v_i^2 + 2ad$$

$$d = \tfrac{1}{2}at^2 + v_i t$$

$$v_f = v_i + at$$

Sample Problem

4. A can is kicked off a cliff that is 19.6 m tall. The horizontal speed given to the can is 12.0 m/sec. Assuming there is no air resistance, how far out from the base of the cliff will the can land?
   A. 12.0 m
   B. 39.2 m
   C. 6.0 m
   D. 24.0 m

Answer

4. D—The problem provides values for the vertical distance, vertical acceleration (i.e., gravity), and the initial vertical speed; therefore the following equation can be transformed to determine the time of flight.

$$d = \tfrac{1}{2}at^2 + v_i t$$

$v_i t$ drops out of the equation because the initial vertical velocity is 0.

$$d = \tfrac{1}{2}at^2$$

Convert the equation to solve for time.

$$t = \sqrt{\dfrac{d}{\tfrac{1}{2}a}}$$

$$t = \sqrt{\dfrac{19.6m}{\tfrac{1}{2}(9.8m/s^2)}}$$

$$t = 2.0 \, sec$$

Once the time of flight is determined is determined, use the following equation to solve for horizontal distance.

$$d_x = v_x t$$

After inserting the appropriate values into the horizontal distance equation, the distance traveled by the can is determined to be 24.0 meters.

$$d_x = v_x t$$

$$d_x = 12 \text{ m/sec} \times 2 \text{ sec}$$

$$d_x = 24 \text{ m}$$

A projectile can also be launched at an angle. This means that the initial velocity of the projectile has two components that make up the motion: horizontal and vertical. Figure 8-1 provides a pictorial representation of the components of the initial speed of an object launched at an angle.

The hypotenuse of the right triangle represents the initial speed (v_i), the legs of the triangle represent the horizontal (v_h) and vertical (v_v) components of the initial speed, and θ represents the angle of the launch. To correctly work with projectile motion, the motion must be clearly separated into the components. One must also remember that both motions occur for the same amount of time. The object will travel horizontally as long as it travels vertically. When attempting to solve projective motion problems, it is best to determine the horizontal and vertical components of the motion before attempting to determine the time of travel of an object. The horizontal and vertical component of the original velocity are represented by the following mathematic equations, where v_i = initial velocity, v_h = the horizontal component of the original velocity, and v_v = the vertical component of the original velocity.

$$v_h = v_i(\cos \theta)$$

$$v_v = v_i(\sin \theta)$$

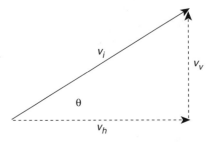

FIGURE 8-1 Components of the initial speed of an object launched at an angle.

Sample Problem

5. A football is thrown with an initial speed of 22.0 m/sec at an angle of 30 degrees with the horizontal. How high does the football rise?
   A. 2.4 m
   B. 4.8 m
   C. 6.2 m
   D. 12.0 m

Answer

5. C—The vertical component of the football's velocity must be determined first using the following equation.

$$v_v = v_i(\sin \theta)$$
$$v_v = 22 \text{ m/sec} \times (\sin 30°)$$
$$v_v = 22 \text{ m/sec} \times 0.5$$
$$v_v = 11 \text{ m/sec}$$

Before we can determine the distance the football rises, we must determine the time of flight of the vertical component using the following formula.

$$v_f = v_i + at$$

Convert the equation to solve for time.

$$t = \frac{v_f - v_i}{a}$$

Remember that acceleration is a result of gravity along the vertical component (y-axis). The initial velocity along the vertical component is 11.0 seconds.

$$t = \frac{0.0 \text{ m/sec} - 11.0 \text{ m/sec}}{-9.8 \text{ m/sec}^2}$$

$$t = 1.12 \text{ sec}$$

Once the vertical components of velocity and time are determined, use the following formula to determine the height the ball rises.

$$d = \tfrac{1}{2}at^2 + v_i t$$

After the appropriate values are inserted into the distance equation, the height the ball rises is determined to be 6.2 m.

$$d = \tfrac{1}{2}at^2 + v_i t$$

$$d = \tfrac{1}{2}(-9.8 \text{ m/sec}^2)(1.12 \text{ sec})^2 + (11.0 \text{ m/sec})(1.12 \text{ sec})$$

$$d = \tfrac{1}{2}(-12.25 \text{ m}) + (12.32 \text{ m})$$

$$d = 6.2 \text{ m}$$

Newton's Laws of Motion

NEWTON'S FIRST LAW OF MOTION

Newton's first law of motion states that a body at rest will remain at rest, and a body in motion will remain in motion, unless acted on by an unbalanced force. Newton's second law of motion states that an unbalanced force will cause acceleration, and this acceleration is directly proportional to the unbalanced force. This relationship is expressed mathematically as follows, where F = force, a = acceleration, and k = the constant of proportionality.

$$F = ka$$

NEWTON'S SECOND LAW OF MOTION

When used in Newton's second law of motion, the constant of proportionality (k) is equal to the mass of the object. Therefore Newton's second law is expressed mathematically as follows, where F = force, m = mass, and a = acceleration.

$$F = ma$$

Sample Problem

6. A box rests on a tabletop. The box has a mass of 25 kg and is acted upon by two forces. The force pushing to the right is 96 N, whereas the force pushing to the left is 180 N. Determine the magnitude of the acceleration of the box.
   A. 11.0 m/sec²
   B. 3.4 m/sec²
   C. 5.5 m/sec²
   D. 7.2 m/sec²

Answer

6. B—To determine the acceleration of the box, it is necessary to first determine the net force acting on the box. Remember that the net force acting on the box is simply the sum of all forces acting on the box. Because the two forces are opposing each other, one force is considered a positive force and the other a negative force. Therefore net force is represented by the following mathematic equation and is determined to be 86 N to the left.

$$\text{NetForce} = F_{left} + (-)F_{right}$$

$$\text{NetForce} = 180\ N + (-)96\ N$$

$$\text{NetForce} = 84\ N \leftarrow$$

Once the net force is determined, use the following equation to determine the magnitude of acceleration of the box.

$$F = ma$$

After the appropriate values are inserted into the force equation, the acceleration of the box is determined to be 3.4 m/sec².

$$F = ma$$

Convert the formula to solve for acceleration.

$$a = \frac{F}{m}$$

$$a = \frac{84\ N}{25\ kg}$$

NOTE: Newtons are also expressed in kg-m/sec².

$$a = 3.4\ m/sec^2$$

If the mass is expressed in kilograms and the acceleration is expressed in meters per second squared (m/sec²), the unit of force is referred to as the *newton* (N). Weight is simply a specialized case of Newton's second law. Weight can be stated mathematically as follows, where *m* = mass in kilograms and *g* = 9.8 m/sec² (i.e., the acceleration associated with gravity).

$$W = mg$$

Sample Problem

7. An object has a mass of 1,250 g. Determine the weight of the object on Earth.
   A. 12,250 N
   B. 122.50 N
   C. 1,225.0 N
   D. 12.25 N

Answer

7. D—To determine the weight of the object on Earth, convert the units of mass to kilograms and apply the following formula.

$$W = mg$$

After the appropriate values are inserted into the weight equation, the weight of the object on Earth is determined to be 12.25 N.

$$W = mg$$

$$W = 1.25\ kg \times 9.8\ m/sec^2$$

$$W = 12.25\ N$$

NEWTON'S THIRD LAW OF MOTION

Newton's third law of motion states that for every action there must be an equal and opposite reaction.

Friction

Friction is a force that opposes motion and is expressed in newtons. If a box (Figure 8-2) is slid on a surface at a constant rate by an applied force, we can deduce that friction is present and is opposing the motion of the box. Because there is no acceleration of the box, it is clear that friction is present and all forces are balanced. This relationship

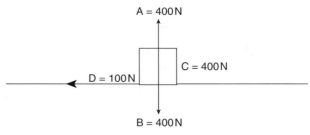

FIGURE 8-2 Depiction of a box being slid on a surface at a constant rate by an applied force.

of balanced forces is represented in the diagram. Note that the normal force *(A)* and the weight *(B)* are balanced. The applied force *(C)* is to the right and has a magnitude of 100 N. The frictional force *(D)* is to the left and must also be 100 N if the box has no acceleration.

Sample Problem

8. A crate is pulled to the right by a rope attached to the crate. The force applied to the rope is 600 N. As the crate slides along the floor, there is a frictional force between the crate and the floor that has a magnitude of 450 N. Determine the magnitude of the net force acting on the crate.
   A. 1,050 N
   B. 600 N
   C. 150 N
   D. 450 N

Answer

8. C—To determine the magnitude of the net force acting on the crate, remember that the magnitude of the net force acting on the box is simply the sum of all forces acting on the box. Because the two forces are opposing each other, applied force to the right and friction to the left, the magnitude of the net force is represented by the following mathematic equation and is determined to be 150 N to the right.

$$\text{NetForce} = F_{right} + (-)F_{left}$$

$$\text{NetForce} = 600 \text{ N} + (-)450 \text{ N}$$

$$\text{NetForce} = 150 \text{ N} \rightarrow$$

Rotation

In addition to displaying linear motion, an object may display a rotating or circular motion. The relationship between the angular displacement and the radius of the circle is expressed mathematically as follows, where θ = the angular displacement, s = arc length, and r = radius of the circle through which the object is moving.

$$\theta = \frac{s}{r}$$

BOX 8-1 **Mathematical Expressions Describing Linear and Rotational Motion**

LINEAR MOTION	ROTATIONAL MOTION
$d = v_{av}t$	$\theta = \omega_{av}t$
$v_f = v_i + at$	$\omega_f = \omega_i + \alpha t$
$d = \frac{1}{2}at^2 + v_i t$	$\theta = \frac{1}{2}\alpha t^2 + \omega_i t$
$v_f^2 = v_i^2 + 2ad$	$\omega_f^2 = \omega_i^2 + 2\alpha\theta$

The average speed of the circular motion can be described by looking at the number of rotations or revolutions an object makes in a given time. The angular speed is the number of radians completed in a given time unit. This is expressed mathematically as follows, where ω = angular speed, θ = the angular displacement, and t = time. When the mathematic expression is considered, it is important to remember that there are 2π radians in one revolution.

$$\omega = \frac{\Delta\theta}{\Delta t}$$

It is also possible to have an angular acceleration as a spinning or rotating object gains or loses speed. This is expressed mathematically as follows, where α = angular acceleration, ω = angular speed, and t = time.

$$\alpha = \frac{\Delta\omega}{\Delta t}$$

The relationship between linear motion and rotational motion is analogous and conforms to Newton's laws. Box 8-1 provides a description of the relationship between the mathematic expressions describing linear motion and those describing rotational motion.

Sample Problem

9. If a bicycle wheel goes from 48 revolutions per second to 84 revolutions per second in 11 seconds, what is the angular acceleration of the wheel?
   A. 3.27 revolutions/sec²
   B. 6.00 revolutions/sec²
   C. 12.0 revolutions/sec²
   D. 1.64 revolutions/sec²

Answer

9. A—To determine the angular acceleration, divide the change in angular speed by the time it took to complete the change in speed.

$$\omega_f = \omega_i + \alpha t$$

Convert the equation to solve for angular acceleration *(a)*.

$$\alpha = \frac{\omega_f - \omega_i}{t}$$

$$\alpha = \frac{84 \text{ rev/sec} - 48 \text{ rev/sec}}{11 \text{ sec}}$$

$$\alpha = 3.27 \text{ rev/sec}^2$$

Uniform Circular Motion

It is possible for an object to experience acceleration even though the object is moving at a constant speed. This is possible because acceleration is a vector quantity and is defined as a change in velocity over a change in time. Velocity has a magnitude and a direction, so even though the speed or magnitude of the velocity is constant, the direction could be changing. In uniform circular motion, this is exactly what is happening. Therefore the object is undergoing an acceleration called a *centripetal acceleration*. Centripetal acceleration is represented mathematically as follows, where a_c = centripetal acceleration, v = the speed of the object in meters per second, and r = the radius of the circle.

$$a_c = \frac{v^2}{r}$$

Because there is a centripetal acceleration, there must also be a centripetal force. Newton's law states that force is a function of mass and acceleration; therefore centripetal force must be a function of mass of an object and centripetal acceleration. This relationship is expressed mathematically as follows, where F_c = centripetal force, m = the mass of the object, v = the velocity, and r = the radius of the circle.

$$F_c = \frac{mv^2}{r}$$

The direction of both the force and the acceleration must be toward the center of the circle. Think of whirling a stone attached to a string in a horizontal circle. The tension in the cord keeps the stone moving in a circular path by pulling inward on the stone.

Sample Problem

10. A 0.6-kg rock is spun in a circle on a 1.2-m string. If the string breaks at 15 N of tension, how fast must the rock be moving?
    A. 30 m/sec
    B. 6 m/sec
    C. 5 m/sec
    D. 5.5 m/sec

Answer

10. D—The centripetal force (15 N) is supplied by the tension in the string. The radius of the circle is 1.2 m, whereas the mass of the rock is 0.6 kg. After these values are inserted in the centripetal force equation, the speed of the stone is determined to be 5.5 m/sec.

$$F_c = \frac{mv^2}{r}$$

Convert the equation to solve for velocity.

$$v = \sqrt{\frac{F_c r}{m}}$$

$$v = \sqrt{\frac{(15 \text{ N})(1.2 \text{ m})}{0.6 \text{ kg}}}$$

$$v = 5.5 \text{ m/sec}$$

Work, Kinetic Energy, and Potential Energy

Work is done when a force is applied and an object moves in the direction of the force. Mathematically this relationship is expressed as follows, where F = force, d = displacement, and θ = the angle between the force and the displacement.

$$W = Fd(\cos \theta)$$

In this equation, force must be expressed in newtons and displacement must be expressed in meters. The angle θ between the force and the displacement is typically 90 degrees, but depending on the nature of the force this angle may be different.

Kinetic energy of an object is the energy resulting from the motion of the object and is represented by the following equation, where *KE* = kinetic energy, *m* = mass of the object, and *v* = velocity.

$$KE = \frac{1}{2}mv^2$$

In this equation, mass must be expressed in kilograms and velocity must be expressed in meters per second.

The potential energy of an object is the energy the object has because of its position and is expressed by the following equation, where *PE* = potential energy, *m* = mass of the object, *g* = acceleration caused by gravity, and *h* = the height at which the object is located above the ground.

$$PE = mgh$$

In this equation, mass must be expressed in kilograms, gravity is a constant expressed as 9.8 m/sec^2, and height is expressed in meters.

Work, kinetic energy, and potential energy are all scalar quantities and are expressed in units called *joules*. A joule is a newton-meter or a kilogram-meter squared per second squared $(\text{kg-m}^2/\text{sec}^2)$. Remember that energy must be conserved; therefore kinetic energy and potential energy can be interchanged if we assume that there is no friction or air resistance present.

Sample Problem

11. A car has a mass of 1,100 kg and is moving at 24 m/sec. How much kinetic energy does the car have as a result of its motion?
    A. 26,400 J
    B. 13,200 J
    C. 633,600 J
    D. 316,800 J

Answer

11. D—The problem provides values for mass and velocity; therefore after the appropriate values for kinetic energy are inserted into the equation, the kinetic energy as a result of the car's motion is determined to be 316,800 J.

$$KE = \frac{1}{2}mv^2$$

$$KE = \frac{1}{2}(1,100 \text{ kg})(24 \text{ m/sec})^2$$

$$KE = 316,800 \text{ J}$$

Linear Momentum and Impulse

Considering Newton's second law of motion in the following slightly different form allows for the development of a new relationship.

$$F = \frac{m\Delta v}{\Delta t}$$

If both sides of this equation are multiplied by Δt, a new relationship between force and time is established and expressed as follows.

$$F\Delta t = m\Delta v$$

The new relationship is referred to as the *impulse equation* because a force applied over a period of time is an impulse. This impulse causes a change in velocity of the object, which results in a change in momentum of the object. *Momentum* is defined as the amount of motion displayed by an object and is represented by the following mathematical equation, where *p* = the momentum in kilograms-meters per second, *m* = the mass in kilograms, and Δ*v* = the change in velocity of the object.

$$P = m\Delta v$$

Momentum is a vector quantity, which means we must have both magnitude and direction to completely express momentum. Momentum must always be conserved, so the momentum before an interaction must equal the momentum after an interaction. This relationship is expressed mathematically as follows.

$$m_1v_1 + m_2v_2' = m_1v_1 + m_2v_2'$$

In this momentum conservation equation, m_1 and m_2 = masses 1 and 2, v_1 and v_2 = the initial velocities of objects 1 and 2, and v_1' and v_2' = the final velocities of objects 1 and 2 after the interaction.

Sample Problem

12. A 30-g rubber ball traveling at 1.60 m/sec strikes a motionless 400-g block of wood. If the ball bounces backward off the block of wood at 1.00 m/sec, how fast will the block of wood be moving?
    A. 0.045 m/sec
    B. 0.195 m/sec
    C. 0.60 m/sec
    D. 1.00 m/sec

Answer

12. A—With the conservation of momentum equation, with the rubber ball established as mass 1 and the block of wood as mass 2, and with the initial velocity of the block of wood being 0, the speed of the block of wood after impact with the ball is determined to be 0.045 m/sec.

$$m_1v_1 + m_2v_2 = m_1v_1' + m_2v_2'$$

Convert the equation to solve for the speed of the block after impact (v_2').

$$v_2' = \frac{m_1v_1 + m_2v_2 - m_1v_1'}{m_2}$$

$$v_2' = \frac{(30\,g \times 1.60\,m/sec) + (400g \times 0\,m/sec) - (30\,g \times 1.0\,m/sec)}{400\,g}$$

$$v_2' = 0.045\,m/sec$$

Universal Gravitation

Newton stated that every object in the universe attracts every other object in the universe. This statement is known as the *law of universal*

gravitation and is expressed mathematically as follows, where F = force of attraction, m_1 and m_2 = the masses of objects 1 and 2 expressed in kilograms, G = the universal gravitation constant $(6.67 \times 10^{-11}\ Nm^2/kg^2)$, and r = the distance between the two objects expressed in meters.

$$F = \frac{Gm_1m_2}{r^2}$$

Sample Problem

13. If object 1 of mass 860 kg is placed 300 m from object 2 of mass 650 kg, what force of attraction exists between the two objects?
    A. 1.24×10^{-7} N
    B. 2.48×10^{-7} N
    C. 4.14×10^{-10} N
    D. 8.28×10^{-10} N

Answer

13. C—When all values are correctly placed in the universal gravitation equation, the force of attraction between the two masses is determined to be 4.14×10^{-10} N.

$$F = \frac{Gm_1m_2}{r^2}$$

$$F = \frac{(6.67 \times 10^{-11}Nm^2/kg^2)(860\ kg)(650\ kg)}{(300\ m)^2}$$

$$F = \frac{0.0000372853\ Nm^2}{90,000\ m^2}$$

$$F = 4.14 \times 10^{-10}N$$

SIMPLE HARMONIC MOTION

An object attached to a spring obeys Hooke's law, which is expressed mathematically as follows.

$$F = -kx$$

In this equation, k is the spring constant and x is the displacement of the spring from its unstrained length. The minus sign indicates that the restoring force always points in a direction opposite that of the displacement of the spring.

Once an object is set into simple harmonic motion, the object oscillates with a maximum displacement known as the *amplitude of the motion*. The energy of the oscillating object takes two distinct forms. The movement of the oscillating object provides kinetic energy, and the stretch or compression of the spring provides potential energy. The potential energy is maximized when the spring has reached maximum amplitude. The kinetic energy is maximized when the spring has returned to the equilibrium position and there is no stretch or compression in the spring. At all other points along the path, both potential energy and kinetic energy are present.

Sample Problem

14. A mass of 1,200 g is placed on a spring, and the spring stretches 85 cm from the equilibrium position. What is the spring constant for this spring?
   A. 138.4 N/cm
   B. 0.14 N/cm
   C. 14.12 N/cm
   D. 1.41 N/cm

Answer

14. B—Before the spring constant is determined, the force must be calculated using Newton's Second Law of Motion. It is important to realize that gravity is providing downward acceleration on the string and that mass must be expressed in units of kilograms.

$$F = ma$$
$$F = 1.2 \text{ kg} \times 9.8 \text{ m/sec}^2$$
$$F = 11.76 \text{ N}$$

After insertion of the appropriate values into the equation for Hooke's law, the spring constant is determined to be 0.14 N/cm.

$$F = -kx$$

Convert the equation to solve for the spring constant (k).

$$-k = \frac{F}{x}$$

$$-k = \frac{11.76 \text{ N}}{85 \text{ cm}}$$

$$-k = 0.14 \text{ N/cm}$$

Waves and Sound

To review waves it is helpful to take a look at the vocabulary associated with waves in Box 8-2.

The frequency of the wave and the period of the wave are inversely related and expressed mathematically as follows, where f = the frequency and T = the period.

$$f = \frac{1}{T}$$

and

$$T = \frac{1}{f}$$

Waves are produced by objects that vibrate or show simple harmonic motion. A wave is a disturbance or pulse that travels through a medium or space. Waves are carriers of energy that travel in the form of light, sound, microwaves, ultraviolet light, x-rays, gamma rays, television, radio, and so on. There are two types of waves, mechanical and electromagnetic.

MECHANICAL WAVES

Each type of mechanical wave is associated with some material or substance called the *medium* for that type. As the wave travels through the medium,

---

BOX 8-2   *Wave Vocabulary*

Crest: High point of a wave.
Trough: Low point of a wave.
Amplitude: Maximum displacement from equilibrium.
Wavelength: Distance between successive identical parts of a wave.
Frequency: Vibrations or oscillations per unit of time. Frequency is expressed in vibrations per second and is measured in hertz (s^{-1}).

the particles that make up the medium undergo displacements of various kinds, depending on the nature of the wave. Examples of these would be sound, water, and seismic.

ELECTROMAGNETIC WAVES

Electromagnetic waves do not require a medium for transmission. These waves are produced by electricity and magnetism and make up the electromagnetic spectrum. These waves all travel at the speed of 3×10^8 m/sec. The components of the electromagnetic spectrum are gamma rays, x-rays, ultraviolet rays, visible light, infrared light, and radio waves.

CLASSIFICATION OF WAVES

Waves are classified by the way they displace matter, or how they cause matter to vibrate. The wave is either transverse or longitudinal in nature. Transverse waves are waves that cause the particles of the medium to vibrate perpendicular to the direction the wave travels. Longitudinal or compressional waves are waves that cause the particles of the medium to vibrate parallel to the direction of the wave. With both longitudinal and transverse waves, the particles of the medium vibrate but *do not* travel with the wave. Longitudinal waves require a medium to be transmitted. The speed at which a wave travels through a medium is determined by the frequency and the wavelength of the wave. This relationship is expressed mathematically as follows, where f = frequency and λ = the wavelength.

$$\text{Speed} = f\lambda$$

The amplitude of a wave is proportional to the potential energy content of the wave. Therefore the higher the wave, the greater the stored energy it is carrying. The higher the frequency, the more kinetic energy the wave possesses, because speed $(v) = f\lambda$ and $KE = \frac{1}{2}mv^2$.

When a string is plucked, a wave will reflect back and forth from one end of the string to the other, creating nodes and antinodes. This is called a *standing wave* because it appears to stand still. Nodes are points along the standing wave that remain stationary. Antinodes are points of maximum energy, where the largest amplitude occurs along the standing wave. The frequency at which

the string vibrates depends on the number of antinodes, the wave speed, and the length of the vibrating string. Mathematically this relationship is expressed as follows.

$$\text{Frequency} = \frac{(\text{Number of antinodes})(\text{Wave speed})}{2(\text{Length})} = \frac{nv}{2L}$$

This relationship is the same for strings that are fixed at both ends and set into vibration, as well as sound waves sent through a pipe open at both ends. However, if sound is sent through a pipe that is closed at one end, the relationship is slightly different and is expressed mathematically as follows.

$$\text{Frequency} = \frac{(\text{Number of antinodes})(\text{Wave speed})}{4(\text{Length})} = \frac{nv}{4L}$$

Antinodes are always formed at open ends, whereas nodes are formed at closed or fixed ends. Remember that the first harmonic or fundamental frequency *(f)* is the lowest frequency at which vibration can occur. Multiples of the fundamental are called *harmonics*. The second harmonic *(2f)* is a frequency that is twice the fundamental. This second harmonic is also called the *first overtone*. The third harmonic *(3f)* is the second overtone, and so on. If a pipe is closed at one end, only the odd harmonics will be present and will have values only of 1, 3, 5, 7, and so on.

Sample Problem

15. A wave in a string travels at 24 m/sec and has a wavelength of 0.90 m. What is the frequency?
    A. 2.67 Hz
    B. 26.67 Hz
    C. 1.33 Hz
    D. 13.33 Hz

Answer

15. B—To determine the frequency of a wave given the speed and wavelength, simply divide the speed of the wave by the wavelength. After insertion of the appropriate values in the following equation, the frequency of the wave is determined to be 26.67 Hz.

$$\text{speed} = f\lambda$$

Convert the equation to solve for frequency *(f)*.

$$f = \frac{speed}{\lambda}$$

$$f = \frac{24 \text{ m/sec}}{0.9 \text{ m}}$$

$$f = 26.67 \text{ Hz}$$

Light

Light is an electromagnetic wave that travels at 3.0×10^8 m/sec. Light needs no medium through which to travel and is a result of electrical and magnetic interactions. We are mainly interested in two properties of light: reflection and refraction.

Reflection is the bouncing back of a wave from a barrier or from a boundary between two media as depicted in Figure 8-3. The law of reflection states that when a wave disturbance is reflected at a boundary of a transmitting medium, the angle of incidence must equal the angle of reflection. The incident wave is the wave that strikes the boundary initially. The reflected wave is the wave that bounces off the boundary. There are terms that should be reviewed as light is studied. A normal line is a line drawn perpendicular to a barrier. The incident wave is the wave that strikes the barrier. The reflected wave is the wave that bounces off and leaves the barrier. The angle of incidence is the angle between the normal and the incident wave. The angle of reflection is the angle between the normal and the reflected wave.

Refraction is the bending of a wave as it passes at an angle from one medium into another if the speed of propagation differs. Different media

have different speeds of propagation, so sound, light, and radio waves travel at different speeds through different media. As waves move from one medium into an optically denser medium, the wave bends toward the normal. As waves move from a medium into an optically less dense medium, the wave bends away from the normal.

The mathematical relationship for this behavior is called *Snell's law*, which is expressed mathematically as follows, where n = the index of refraction and θ = the angle of refraction.

$$n_1 \sin\theta_1 = n_2 \sin\theta_2$$

The index of refraction is a ratio of the speed of light in a vacuum to the speed of light in a given material. This mathematic relationship is expressed as follows, where c = the speed of light in a vacuum (3×10^8 m/sec) and v_s = the speed of light in a given substance.

$$n = \frac{c}{v_s}$$

Sample Problem

16. If the index of refraction for quartz is 1.46, what is the speed of light in quartz?
    A. 2.05×10^8 m/sec
    B. 4.38×10^8 m/sec
    C. 1.25×10^8 m/sec
    D. 0.489×10^8 m/sec

Answer

16. A—To determine the speed of light in quartz, divide the speed of light by index of refraction for quartz. Through use of the following equation, the speed of light in quartz is determined to be 2.05×10^8 m/sec.

$$n = \frac{c}{v_s}$$

Convert the equation to solve for speed of light in a substance (v_s).

$$v_s = \frac{3 \times 10^8 \text{ m/sec}}{1.46}$$

$$v_s = 2.05 \times 10^8 \text{ m/sec}$$

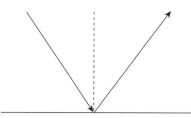

FIGURE 8-3   Reflection is a wave bouncing back from a barrier or from a boundary between two media.

Optics

Mirrors are of two types: concave and convex. Concave mirrors have positive focal lengths, whereas convex mirrors have negative focal lengths. Concave mirrors form a variety of image shapes, sizes, and orientations depending on the focal length of the mirror and where the object is placed. With the object beyond the center of curvature (C), we have an image that is smaller than the object and inverted in orientation. If we place the object at C, the resulting image is the same size as the object and inverted in orientation. If the object is between C and the focal point (f), the image is larger than the object and inverted in orientation. If the object is at f, there is no image formed. If the object is between f and the mirror, the image is upright and larger in size. Convex mirrors can form only images that are smaller and upright. Real images are always inverted, and virtual images are always upright. The mathematic relationship between the object distance (d_o), image distance (d_i), and focal length (f) is expressed as follows.

$$\frac{1}{d_o} + \frac{1}{d_i} = \frac{1}{f}$$

Lenses form images by refraction. There are two basic types of lenses: convex (converging) and concave (diverging). Convex lenses always have positive focal lengths, and concave lenses always have negative focal lengths. Convex lenses can form a variety of image shapes, sizes, and orientations depending on the focal length of the lens and the object's position. When an object is placed at a position greater than 2f, the image is reduced, inverted, and on the opposite side of the lens. The placement of an object at 2f results in an image that is the same size as the object, inverted, and on the opposite side of the lens. The placement of an object between 2f and f results in an image that is larger than the object, inverted, and on the opposite side of the lens. When the object is placed at f, no image is formed. If the object is between f and the lens, the image is upright, larger, and on the same side of the lens. A concave lens can form only an image that is upright and smaller than the object.

17. A concave mirror has a focal length of 15 cm. If an object is placed at 30 cm, what is the image distance?
    A. 10 cm
    B. 15 cm
    C. 30 cm
    D. 20 cm

Answer

17. C—The image distance is determined by subtracting the inverse of the object distance from the inverse of the focal length and taking the reciprocal of the result. After insertion of the appropriate values in the equation, it is determined that the image distance is 30 cm.

$$\frac{1}{d_o} + \frac{1}{d_i} = \frac{1}{f}$$

Convert the equation to solve for image distance (d_i).

$$\frac{1}{d_i} = \frac{1}{f} - \frac{1}{d_o}$$

$$\frac{1}{d_i} = \frac{1}{15 \text{ cm}} - \frac{1}{30 \text{ cm}}$$

$$\frac{1}{d_i} = \frac{2}{30 \text{ cm}} - \frac{1}{30 \text{ cm}}$$

$$\frac{1}{d_i} = \frac{1}{30 \text{ cm}}$$

Take the reciprocal of $\frac{1}{d_i}$ to determine the image distance.

$$d_i = 30 \text{ cm}$$

Static Electricity and Coulomb's Law

There are two types of basic charge: positive (protons) and negative (electrons). Like charges repel, whereas opposite charges attract. The unit of charge is the coulomb. The force of attraction or repulsion is determined by the mathematic relationship expressed by Coulomb's law, where k = a constant (9×10^9 N-m^2/C^2), q_1 and q_2 = the charges on objects 1 and 2 expressed in coulombs, and r = the distance between the two charged objects in meters.

$$F = \frac{k\,q_1 q_2}{r^2}$$

Sample Problem

18. An object of charge 16 μC is placed 50 cm from an object of charge 30 μC. What is the magnitude of the resulting force between the two objects?
    A. 17.28 N
    B. 8.64 N
    C. 1.73 × 10^{13} N
    D. 8.64 × 10^{12} N

Answer

18. A—To solve this problem use Coulomb's law, remembering that 1 μC is 1×10^{-6} C, and convert the distance to meters. After insertion of the correct values into the equation, remembering to square the distance, the force between the two objects is determined to be 17.28 N.

$$F = \frac{k\,q_1 q_2}{r^2}$$

$$F = \frac{\left(9 \times 10^9 \text{ Nm}^2/\text{C}^2\right)\left(16 \times 10^{-6} \text{ C}\right)\left(30 \times 10^{-6} \text{ C}\right)}{\left(0.5 \text{ m}\right)^2}$$

$$F = \frac{\left(9 \times 10^9 \text{ Nm}^2/\text{C}^2\right)\left(16 \times 10^{-6} \text{ C}\right)\left(30 \times 10^{-6} \text{ C}\right)}{\left(0.5 \text{ m}\right)^2}$$

$$F = 17.28 \text{ N}$$

Electric Fields

An electric field exists around charged objects. This field interacts with a positive test charge. If the electric field is generated by a negative charge, a test charge would experience an attractive force. If the electric field is generated by a positive charge, a test charge would experience a repulsive force. Owing to these interactions, scientists have defined the direction of an electric field to be away from a positive charge and toward a negative charge. The magnitude of an electric field is stated mathematically as follows, where E = the magnitude of the electric field, F = the force a test charge would experience and q_o = the magnitude of the test charge.

$$E = \frac{F}{q_o}$$

It is also possible to determine the electric field surrounding point charge by using the following mathematic expression:

$$E = \frac{kq}{r^2}$$

Because electric fields are vector quantities, they should be treated as such.

Sample Problem

19. An electric field of magnitude 280,000 N/C points due east at a certain spot. What are the magnitude and direction of the force that acts on a charge of −10 μC?
    A. 2.8 N to the west
    B. 2.8 N to the east
    C. 28 N to the west
    D. 28 N to the east

Answer

19. A—To determine the magnitude of the force acting on the charge, multiply the magnitude of the electric field by the magnitude of the test charge. Because the charge is negative, it acts opposite to the direction of the electric field. After insertion of the appropriate values in the electric field equation, the magnitude of the charge is determined to be 2.8 N to the west.

$$E = \frac{F}{q_o}$$

Convert the equation to solve for the force the test charge will experience (F).

$$F = Eq_o$$

$$F = (280{,}000 \text{ N/C}) \, (-10 \text{ μC})$$

Remember that 1 μC is 1×10^{-6} C.

$$F = (280{,}000 \text{ N/C}) (-10 \text{ μC})$$

$$F = (280{,}000 \text{ N/C})(-0.00001 \text{ C})$$

$$F = -2.8 \text{ N}$$

The negative sign in the answer indicates the direction of the force relative to the electric field.

$$F = 2.8 \text{ N to the west}$$

DC CIRCUITS

The flow of current is determined by the voltage available and the resistance of the circuit. The mathematic relationship between voltage and resistance is known as *Ohm's law* and is expressed as follows, where V = potential difference in voltage expressed in volts, I = current expressed in amperes, and R = resistance expressed in ohms.

$$V = IR$$

There are two types of basic circuits. A series circuit has only one pathway through which current can flow, so current is the same through all resistors. A parallel circuit has several pathways through which current can flow, but all resistors are connected directly to the same battery, so the voltage supplied for each resistor is the same. To determine the total resistance of a series circuit, you would add the individual resistors. To determine the total resistance of a parallel circuit, you would add the reciprocal of the individual resistors and then take the reciprocal of that value. Once the total resistance is determined and the type of circuit used is known, the current flowing through each resistor can be determined.

Sample Problem

20. A circuit consists of a 10-ohm resistor, a 15-ohm resistor, and a 25-ohm resistor. The resistors are placed in series and then wired to a 100-V power supply. Determine the current flowing in the circuit.
    A. 0.5 amp
    B. 2.0 amp
    C. 10.0 amp
    D. 4.0 amp

Answer

20. B—Before the current flowing through the circuit is determined, the total resistance must be calculated. Because the resistors are placed in a series, the total resistance is determined by adding the individual values of the individual resistors.

$$\text{Total Resistance}_{(\text{in a series})} = R_1 + R_2 + R_3$$

$$\text{Total Resistance}_{(\text{in a series})} = 10 \text{ ohm} + 15 \text{ ohm} + 25 \text{ ohm}$$

$$\text{Total Resistance}_{(\text{in a series})} = 50 \text{ ohm}$$

To determine the current in the circuit, use the Ohm's law equation. After insertion of the appropriate values into the equation, the current flowing in the circuit is determined to be 2.0 amp.

$$V = IR$$

Convert the equation to solve for current *(I)*.

$$I = \frac{100 \text{ volts}}{50 \text{ ohms}}$$

$$I = 2.0 \text{ amps}$$

Workspace

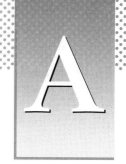

MATHEMATICS PRACTICE TEST

1. What kind of number system is commonly used in the United States?
   A. Tertiary
   B. Decimal
   C. Napoleonic
   D. Binary

2. Place value is not used in which numeric system?
   A. Arabian
   B. Cyrillic
   C. Decimal
   D. Roman

3. The numeral 0 is not used in which numeric system?
   A. Roman
   B. Decimal
   C. Chinese
   D. Bulgarian

4. A telemarketer must call 157 U.S. phone numbers every shift to meet their quota. How many buttons will have to be pushed to make 157 long-distance calls?
   A. 2,000
   B. 1,727
   C. 1,099
   D. 1,570

5. A newborn weighs 3,459 grams. There are 453.59 grams per pound. What is the infant's weight in pounds and ounces?
   A. 7 lb 10 oz
   B. 10 lb 7 oz
   C. 13 lb 3 oz
   D. 3 lb 13 oz

6. What temperature in Celsius is 98.6° Fahrenheit? (Enter numeric value only. If rounding is necessary round to the whole number.) _____

7. A nurse works in a military hospital from 1300 to 2000. What time of day does this nurse work?
   A. Early morning to early afternoon
   B. Lunch time to midnight
   C. Early afternoon to bedtime
   D. Midnight to sunrise

8. A nurse is reviewing the daily intake and output (I&O) of a patient consuming a clear diet. The drainage bag denotes a total of 1,000 mL for the past 24 hours. The total intake is:
   2 8oz cups of coffee
   1 16-oz serving of clear soup
   1 pint of water consumed throughout the day
   How much is the deficit in milliliters? (Enter numeric value only. If rounding is necessary round to the whole number.)
   _____

9. A woman received a bottle of perfume as a present. The bottle contains $1/2$ oz of perfume. How many milliliters is this? (Enter numeric value only. If rounding is necessary round to the whole number.)
   _____

10. The metric system of measurement was developed in France during Napoleon's reign. It is based on what multiplication factor?
    A. The length of Napoleon's forearm
    B. 2
    C. 10
    D. Atomic weight of helium

11. How many meters are in a kilometer? (Enter numeric value only.) _____

12. How many grams are in a kilogram? (Enter numeric value only.) _____

13. To convert pounds to kilograms, what factor is used?
    A. 2.2
    B. 0.334
    C. 10
    D. 22

14. A teacher's aide is preparing a snack for the class. In order to prepare the powdered drink, the aide must convert the directions to metric. The directions say, "Dilute contents of package in 2 quarts of water." The aide has a measuring device marked in liters. How many liters of water should be used? (Enter numeric value only. If rounding is required, round to the nearest tenth.) _____

15. How many milliliters are in 1 liter?
    A. 30
    B. 10
    C. 100
    D. 1,000

16. A seamstress is measuring a model for a new dress. The tape measure is marked in centimeters. The seamstress needs to convert that measurement into inches. If the model's waist measurement is 65.4 centimeters, what is that in inches?
    A. 25.74 inches
    B. 166.12 inches
    C. 32.50 inches
    D. 17 inches

17. There are 2.54 centimeters in an inch. How many centimeters are in 1 foot? (Enter numeric value only. If rounding is necessary round to the whole number.) _____

18. How many centimeters in a millimeter?
    A. $1/10$
    B. 1
    C. 10
    D. 100

19. How many centimeters in a meter?
    A. $1/100$
    B. 10
    C. 100
    D. 1,000

20. A newspaper kiosk sells 10 varieties of newspapers from around the world. The average daily sales for some of the varieties are as follows:
    English language newspapers—eight papers, sells 25 of each paper each day
    French language newspapers—two papers, sells one of each paper each day
    Korean language newspapers—one paper, sells 16 each day
    Japanese language newspapers—eight papers, sells 16 of each paper each day
    Russian language newspapers—one paper, sells 22 each day
    How many of these newspapers are sold each day? (Enter numeric value only. If rounding is necessary round to the whole number.) _____

21. A hospital day staff consists of 25 registered nurses, 75 unlicensed assistants, five phlebologists, six receptionists and office staff, and 45 physicians. One summer day the staff was at only 68% strength. How many people were working that day? (Enter numeric value only. If rounding is necessary round to the whole number.) _____

22. A farmer raises chickens for eggs and meat. Any chicken that does not lay at least one egg a week is moved to the slaughterhouse. The farmer has 765 chickens that can lay one egg each day. Each day 80% of the chickens lay eggs. How many eggs does the farmer collect each day? (Enter numeric value only. If rounding is necessary round to the whole number.) _____

23. Last night at the hospital 76 babies were born. Of the births, 45% were girls. How many boys were born last night? (Enter numeric value only. If rounding is necessary round to the whole number.) _____

24. The doctor tells the patient to cut back on coffee. The patient usually has four 8-oz cups of coffee per day. If the doctor told him to cut back by 25%, how many ounces of coffee can the patient have each day? (Enter numeric value only. If rounding is necessary round to the whole number.) _____

25. Ratio and proportion:
    0.8:10 :: x:100
    A. x = 0.8
    B. x = 8
    C. x = 80
    D. x = 800

26. Add: 9.98 + 0.065 =
    A. 10.63
    B. 10.045
    C. 1.0063
    D. 998.065

27. Add: 6 + 12.55 + 5.022 =
    A. 18.55
    B. 23.572
    C. 30.025
    D. 16.475

28. Add: 23.5 + 7.025 =
    A. 30.525
    B. 30.5
    C. 30.025
    D. 16.475

29. Subtract: 32.21 – 4.68 =
    A. 14.59
    B. 27.53
    C. 1.459
    D. 31.742

30. Subtract: 15.7 – 9.8 =
    A. 6.1
    B. 8.96
    C. 5.9
    D. 4.30

31. Subtract: 10.012 – 0.120 =
    A. 10
    B. 9.012
    C. 10.122
    D. 9.892

32. Multiply: (7.2)(0.34) =
    A. 14.12
    B. 0.234
    C. 7.64
    D. 2.448

33. Multiply: (99)(0.56) =
    A. 99.30
    B. 99.56
    C. 55.44
    D. 199.54

34. Multiply: (88)(7.08) =
    A. 862.5
    B. 88.040
    C. 64.252
    D. 623.04

35. Multiply: 375 × 2.3 =
    A. 862.5
    B. 750
    C. 225.75
    D. 1125

36. How many gallons are in 48 fluid ounces?
    A. 0.25 gallons
    B. 0.75 gallons
    C. 0.48 gallons
    D. 0.375 gallons

37. A shopper spends $75.64 at one store and $22.43 at the next store. The shopper started out with $100.00. How much money does the shopper have left?
    A. $1.93
    B. $5.00
    C. $0.72
    D. $20.13

38. A worker is filling out his timesheet. He worked 8 hours on Monday, 7 hours and 30 minutes on Tuesday, 8¾ hours on Wednesday, 4 hours on Thursday, and 8¼ hours on Friday. If he earns $14.35 per hour, what will be his gross pay for this week? (Enter numeric value only.)

    _____

39. A farmer counts his flock of chickens. He has five red chickens, 17 white chickens, three black chickens, and one spotted chicken in his flock. What is the percentage of white chickens in the flock? (Enter numeric value only. If rounding is necessary round to the whole number.) _____

40. What number in Arabic numerals is Roman numeral MCMXLIV? (Enter numeric value only.) _____

Mathematics Answer Key

1. B
2. D
3. A
4. B
5. A
6. 37
7. C
8. 440
9. 15
10. C
11. 1,000
12. 1,000
13. A
14. 1.9
15. D
16. A
17. 30.48
18. A
19. C
20. 368

21. 106
22. 612
23. 42
24. 24
25. B
26. B
27. B
28. A
29. B
30. C
31. D
32. D
33. C
34. D
35. A
36. D
37. A
38. 523.78
39. 65
40. 1,944

READING COMPREHENSION PRACTICE TEST

Blood Pressure

Lub-dub! Lub-dub! Lub-dub! This sound is made by the rapid contracting and extending of the chamber doors on the inside of the heart. This ventricular contracting injects roughly 70 milliliters of blood into a vascular system with a given volume at differing pressure.

Blood pressure refers to the pressure in the arterial system and is typically taken in the brachial artery of the arm, because the pressure at different places along the circulatory route is different. Blood pressure is simply the force that the blood exerts in all directions within any given area and is the basis for the movement of blood from the heart, through the body, and back to the heart. This pressure is commonly expressed as a ratio of the systolic pressure over the diastolic pressure.

The systolic pressure or "high peak" pressure takes place within the arterial system as ventricles contract and force blood into the arteries. The diastolic pressure or "low peak" pressure takes place within this arterial system just before the next ventricular contraction.

An increase in blood pressure can occur if the arterial walls lose some of their elasticity with age or disease.

1. What is the main idea of the passage?
   A. Blood pressure overall measures the elasticity of the arteries near the heart as they stretch to accommodate expelled blood.
   B. Blood pressure within the arterial system takes into account that pressure is different at varying locations.
   C. Blood pressure is simply the force that the blood exerts in all directions within any given area, measured as a ratio.
   D. Blood pressure represents the pulse difference between ventricular contractions.

2. Which statement is not a detail from the passage?
   A. The ventricular contraction asserts capillary pressure that is about 70 mm Hg.
   B. The pressures at different places in the circulatory system are different.
   C. Increase in blood pressure can occur if arterial walls lose some of their elasticity.
   D. Blood pressure is expressed as a ratio of systolic over diastolic pressure.

3. What is the meaning of the word *elasticity* in the last paragraph?
   A. Something that is able to resist and be flexible
   B. Something that is like plastic
   C. Something that is dynamic and electrifying
   D. Something that is silly

4. What is the author's primary purpose in writing this essay?
   A. To entertain
   B. To analyze
   C. To inform
   D. To persuade

Blood Pressure Regulators

The body is composed of systems that have evolved and diversified in order to maintain the natural functions and processes they regulate. One such system that has these regulators is the body's cardiovascular system. The body's pump, which regulates the flow of vitally needed oxygen to all cells of the body as well as the discard of carbon dioxide and other waste products, is the heart.

Because blood pressure varies at different points within the body, differing components are needed to keep the body's blood pressure regulated. Three of the basic components are baroreceptors, chemoreceptors, and the kidneys.

Baroreceptors are stretch receptors composed of fine branching nerve endings and are contained along the walls of the arteries near the heart and in other areas of the body as well. Impulses are related to this stretching along the arterial walls, which causes these baroreceptors to send out even more impulses to the heart, arteries, and veins, causing the blood pressure to go either up or down.

Chemoreceptors are located along the walls of the arteries and monitor changes in oxygen level, carbon dioxide, and pH. Just think! A fall in oxygen causes receptors to send impulses to raise the blood pressure.

The kidneys play a role in regulating blood pressure by absorbing salts and water and removing wastes.

Hormones secreted by the adrenal cortex cause the kidney to keep or let go of any salt and water. This has an influence on blood volume and consequently on blood pressure.

5. What is the main idea of the passage?
   A. Blood pressure can be treated only by monitoring baroreceptors.
   B. Blood pressure can be treated only by monitoring chemoreceptors.
   C. Blood pressure can be treated only by monitoring the kidneys.
   D. Blood pressure can be regulated through baroreceptors, chemoreceptors, and the kidneys.

6. Which statement is not a detail from the passage?
   A. Baroreceptors are rigid and static nerve endings that are contained along the arterial walls and send out messages along the nerve pathway.
   B. Chemoreceptors are located along the walls of the arteries and monitor changes in oxygen level.
   C. The kidneys play a role in regulating blood pressure by absorbing salts and water.
   D. The heart is the body's pump, which regulates the flow of vitally needed oxygen to cells of the body.

7. What is the meaning of the word *evolved* in the first paragraph?
   A. To spread
   B. To gradually develop
   C. To revolve
   D. To shift

8. What is the writer's primary purpose in writing this essay?
   A. To analyze
   B. To inform
   C. To entertain
   D. To persuade

Doppler Effect

Have you ever wondered why the whistle of a traveling, distant locomotive predicts its approach several yards before anyone actually sees it? Or why an oncoming ambulance's screaming siren is heard momentarily several feet before the ambulance comes into full view, before it passes you, and why its siren is still heard faintly well after the ambulance is out of sight?

What you are witnessing is a scientific phenomenon known as the *Doppler effect*. What takes place is truly remarkable. In both of these instances, when the train or ambulance moves toward the sound waves in front of it, the sound waves are pulled closer together and have a higher frequency. In either instance the listener positioned in front of the moving object hears a higher pitch. The ambulance and locomotive are progressively moving away from the sound waves behind them, causing the waves to be farther apart and to have a lower frequency. These fast-approaching modes of transportation distance themselves past the listener, who hears a lower pitch.

9. Which statement is not listed as a detail in the passage?
   A. The oncoming sound waves have a higher pitch owing to high frequency and closeness of waves.
   B. The oncoming sound waves have a higher pitch owing to low frequency and closeness of waves.
   C. The whistling sound of the locomotive as it approaches and passes can be explained by the Doppler effect.
   D. The high-pitched sound of the ambulance as it approaches and passes can be explained by the Doppler effect.

10. What is the main idea of the passage?
    A. Trains and ambulances make distinctly loud noises.
    B. Low-frequency waves make high-pitched sounds.
    C. High-frequency waves make low-pitched sounds.
    D. The Doppler effect explains the rationale for why the sound is heard initially more strongly and then faintly after a moving object has passed.

11. What is the meaning of the word *phenomenon* in the second paragraph?
    A. Something that is lifeless to the senses
    B. Something that is nonchalant
    C. Something that is significant but unusual
    D. Something that is chemical in origin

12. What is the author's primary purpose in writing this essay?
    A. To entertain
    B. To inform
    C. To analyze
    D. To persuade

Electrocardiogram

Beep!... Beep!... Beep! is the audible rhythmic sound made as the strength of the heart muscle is measured. The signal cadence has a characteristic record that varies in every individual. This record is called an *electrocardiogram*, or ECG.

In the body an array of systemic neural responses constantly occur, sending out electrical currents. The electrical currents can be detected on the surface of the body, and if a person is hooked to an amplifier, these impulses are recorded by an electrocardiograph.

Most of the information obtained is about the heart because the heart sends out electrical currents in waves. This "wave of excitation" emitted spreads through the heart wall and is accompanied by electrical changes. The wave takes place in three distinct steps.

Initially the wave of excitation accompanied by an electrical change lasts for approximately 1 to 2 seconds after contraction of the cardiac muscle. The electrical impulses are discharged rhythmically from the sinoatrial (SA) node, the pacemaker of the heart. This spread of excitation over the muscle of the atrium indicates that the atrium has contracted.

Next, the peak of the ECG reading is due to the atrioventricular or AV node causing the ventricle to become excited.

Finally, the ventricles relax, and any changes in the wave indicate to trained medical staff any abnormalities within the heart.

13. What is the author's primary purpose in writing the essay?
    A. To persuade
    B. To entertain
    C. To inform
    D. To analyze

14. Which statement is not listed as a detail within the passage?
    A. Changes in the ECG are typically used for diagnosis of abnormal cardiac rhythm.
    B. The signal has a characteristic record called the *electrocardiogram*.
    C. The wave of excitation starts at the SA node.
    D. The wave of excitation spreads through the heart wall and is accompanied by electrical changes.

15. What is the meaning of the word *emitted* as it is used in the second paragraph?
    A. Repelled
    B. Released
    C. Closed
    D. Charged

16. What is the main idea of the passage?
    A. Electrical currents within the body are due to electrostatic charges set off by the heart.
    B. The electrocardiogram systematically and rather quickly measures the stages at which the wave of excitation occurs within the heart and records it.
    C. The wave of excitation is detected on the surface of the body and measures the atrial excitation of the heart.
    D. The electrical currents within the body are in direct relation to the wave of excitation measured by the electrocardiogram.

The Water Cycle

Water is needed to sustain practically all life functions on planet Earth. A single drop of this compound is composed of an oxygen atom that shares its electrons with each of the two hydrogen atoms.

The cycle starts when precipitation such as rain, snow, sleet, or hail descends from the sky onto the ground. Water not absorbed immediately from the precipitation is known as *runoff*. The runoff flows across the land and collects in groundwater reservoirs, rivers, streams, and oceans.

Evaporation takes place when liquid water changes into water vapor, which is a gas. Water vapor returns to the air from surface water and plants.

Ultimately, condensation happens when this water vapor cools and changes back into droplets of liquid. In fact, the puffy, cotton clouds that we observe are formed by condensation. When the clouds become heavily laden with liquid droplets, precipitation ensues.

17. What is the meaning of the word *composed* in the first paragraph?
    A. To consist of
    B. To be uniquely discovered
    C. To be set apart
    D. To be surprised

18. What is the main idea of this passage?
    A. The formation of water from the joining of two hydrogen atoms to one atom of oxygen
    B. The versatility and importance of water as a universal solvent
    C. The explanation of the different components of the water cycle
    D. Rain is a trivial part of the life cycle.

19. Which statement is not a detail from the passage?
    A. A single drop of water is made of a couple of hydrogen atoms and oxygen atoms.
    B. Evaporation takes place when liquid water changes into water vapor.
    C. Water not absorbed is runoff.
    D. Condensation fails to happen when water vapor cools and changes back into droplets of liquid.

20. What was the author's primary purpose for writing this essay?
    A. To entertain
    B. To persuade
    C. To analyze
    D. To inform

Reading Comprehension Answer Key

1. C
2. A
3. A
4. C
5. D
6. A
7. B
8. B
9. B
10. D

11. C
12. B
13. C
14. A
15. B
16. B
17. A
18. C
19. D
20. D

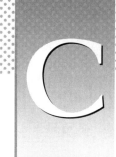

GRAMMAR AND VOCABULARY PRACTICE TEST

1. Which sentence is grammatically correct?
    A. The little girl wanted he to read a story to her.
    B. The little girl wanted his to read a story to her.
    C. The little girl wanted him to read a story to her.
    D. The little girl wanted himself to read a story to her.

2. Select the word or phrase that will make the sentence grammatically correct.
    Within the _____ of the hospital, great emphasis is placed on calmness.
    A. cafeteria
    B. milieu
    C. metabolism
    D. component

3. What is the best description for the term *quotient*?
    A. The minimum number of members needed to be present for a vote to be valid
    B. The protocol used when a sterile field must be maintained
    C. A math term naming the answer in a division question
    D. The preferred inoculation site for a newborn infant

4. Select the word or phrase that will make the sentence grammatically correct.
    The nurse has a _____ to the *Journal of Nursing Education*.
    A. subscription
    B. prescription
    C. recipe
    D. receipt

5. Which statement uses a euphemism?
    A. The fireman bravely entered the burning building.
    B. The nurse told the family, "I'm sorry, your father has passed away."
    C. The orderly was laughing about the patient's vomiting episode.
    D. Her husband was overjoyed when she told him she was pregnant.

6. Select the word or phrase that will identify the correct meaning of the underlined word.
    <u>Progeny</u> is a term used to describe a person's _____.
    A. creditors
    B. offspring
    C. hereditary disease
    D. health status

7. Select the meaning of the underlined word in the sentence.
    The <u>proliferation</u> of resistant bacteria has alarmed medical professionals.
    A. Increase
    B. Reduction
    C. Strength
    D. Appearance

8. What is the best description for the word *laceration*?
    A. The means by which nursing mothers produce milk for their babies
    B. A deep, ragged tear
    C. A medical term used to describe the removal of the tear ducts
    D. An intolerance of dairy products

9. Select the sentence that is grammatically correct.
    A. The nurse spoke to my sister and I about our mother's condition.
    B. The nurse spoke to my sister and me about our mother's condition.
    C. The nurse spoke to me and my sister about our mother's condition.
    D. The nurse spoke to I and my sister about our mother's condition.

10. The nurse noted in the chart, "The patient is lethargic." How was the patient behaving?
    A. Pacing the halls, yelling at the staff
    B. Difficult to arouse
    C. Shaking uncontrollably
    D. Not responding to painful stimuli

11. What is the best description for the word *contraction*?
    A. Spasm
    B. Decrease
    C. Treaty
    D. Moderate

12. What is another word for *skull?*
    A. Spine
    B. Ability
    C. Cranium
    D. Zygote

13. Select the meaning of the underlined word in the sentence.
    In medicine, the <u>desired</u> outcome is recovery.
    A. expectation
    B. analysis
    C. wished for
    D. diagnosis

14. Select the word or phrase that makes this sentence grammatically correct.
    She has always been afraid of _____ to the doctor.
    A. have gone
    B. going
    C. to go
    D. go

15. What is the best description for the word *distal?*
    A. The part of the heart that receives blood from the lungs
    B. Urgent
    C. The part of the body farthest from the injury
    D. Empathetic

16. What is the best description for the term *triage?*
    A. The stand with three legs used to support an IV pump
    B. The order in which patients are to be treated
    C. The physician's prescription for a drug to be taken three times a day
    D. The shift for nursing duty beginning at 3 PM and ending at 11 PM

17. Select the word or phrase that makes this sentence grammatically correct.
    I want _____ to sing.
    A. he
    B. his
    C. him
    D. himself

18. Which word means "the thickness of a liquid"?
    A. Viscosity
    B. Zygote
    C. Sublingual
    D. Adhesion

19. Select the meaning of the underlined word in the sentence.
    The client's condition was <u>exacerbated</u> in the fall.
    A. Improved
    B. Made worse
    C. Eliminated
    D. Created a scar

20. Select the meaning of the underlined word in the sentence.
    His skin was unevenly <u>pigmented</u> by the disease.
    A. Scarred
    B. Spotted
    C. Broken
    D. Colored

21. Select the word or phrase that will make the sentence grammatically correct.
    The patient asked the doctor to help him complete the _____ needed to approve the surgery.
    A. from
    B. form
    C. pillow
    D. syringe

22. Select the meaning of the underlined word in the sentence.
    His <u>metabolism</u> could not tolerate the new medication.
    A. Digestive system
    B. Processing reaction
    C. Respiratory rate
    D. Obesity

23. Select the word or phrase that makes this sentence grammatically correct.
    She has lived in Texas _____ she was a child.
    A. since
    B. for
    C. from
    D. during

24. What is the best description for the term *combination*?
    A. Putting two or more things together
    B. The beginning of a fire
    C. The reason for an action
    D. The change seen when a drug is administered

25. What is the best description for the term *febrile*?
    A. Mental incompetence
    B. Having a fever
    C. Pregnant
    D. Having clogged sinuses

26. Select the meaning of the underlined word in the sentence.
    The medication will make the patient <u>photosensitive</u>.
    A. Unable to eat citrus fruit
    B. Easily burned when in direct sunlight
    C. Nauseated
    D. Impotent

27. Select the word or phrase that makes this sentence grammatically correct.
    She had to choose _____ five dresses for the party.
    A. after
    B. among
    C. between
    D. before

28. Select the meaning of the underlined word in the sentence.
    The nurse was keeping careful watch on the patient's <u>respiration</u>.
    A. Breathing
    B. Skin color
    C. Pulse
    D. Diet

29. Select the meaning of the underlined word in the sentence.
    The nurse must <u>assess</u> the patient's symptoms.
    A. Choose the most life-threatening of
    B. Report to the health care provider about
    C. Observe and make note of
    D. Eliminate

30. Select the meaning of the underlined word in the sentence.
    The nurse discussed the <u>diet plan</u> with the patient.
    A. Regime
    B. Regimen
    C. Supposition
    D. Substitution

31. Select the meaning of the underlined word in the sentence.
    The nurse gave instructions to the patient on the care of his <u>renal</u> disease.
    A. Fatal
    B. Kidney
    C. Heart
    D. Lung

32. Which sentence is grammatically correct?
    A. She put the carton of milk into the refrigerator.
    B. Her put the carton of milk into the refrigerator.
    C. Herself put the carton of milk into the refrigerator.
    D. Ours put the carton of milk into the refrigerator.

33. Select the word or phrase that makes this sentence grammatically correct.
    Every morning after a shower, I shave _____.
    A. me
    B. myself
    C. mine
    D. my

34. Select the meaning of the underlined word in the sentence.
    The medication was given <u>sublingually</u>.
    A. Under the eyelid
    B. Under the tongue
    C. By nasal inhaler
    D. By injection

35. Select the meaning of the underlined word in the sentence.
    The patient went into <u>spasm</u>.
    A. Unconsciousness
    B. Convulsion
    C. Coronary arrest
    D. Remission

36. When a circuit is completed, what has been finished?
    A. Lap
    B. Test
    C. Diagnosis
    D. Round shape

37. Select the meaning of the underlined word in the sentence.
    The prescription called for administration of the medication q.i.d.
    A. Once daily
    B. Four times a day
    C. Every 8 hours
    D. At bedtime

38. Select the word or phrase that will make the sentence grammatically correct.
    It is always a good idea to _____ any exam.
    A. answer
    B. rest on
    C. prepare for
    D. cram

39. Select the meaning of the underlined word in the sentence.
    When examined, the laboring mother was at 50% dilation.
    A. Blood pressure
    B. Cervical opening
    C. Birth process
    D. Exhumation

40. Select the meaning of the underlined word in the sentence.
    The doctor made an initial examination of the patient.
    A. Complete
    B. First
    C. Incomplete
    D. Discharge

41. What is the best description for the term fracture?
    A. Break
    B. Brake
    C. Cut
    D. Cure

42. To implement something is to _____.
    A. prevent it from occurring
    B. emphasize the importance of
    C. cause it to happen
    D. follow from beginning to end

43. Select the meaning of the underlined word in the sentence.
    The results of the poll were not valid because the sample size was not large enough.
    A. Applicable
    B. Obtainable
    C. Presentable
    D. Factual

44. Select the word or phrase in the sentence that is not used correctly.
    People of similar linguistic, culture, or religious backgrounds tend to locate each other at international gatherings.
    A. of
    B. culture
    C. to locate
    D. each other

45. Posterior refers to which part of the body?
    A. Topmost
    B. Lowermost
    C. Front
    D. Back

46. Select the word or phrase that makes this sentence grammatically correct.
    He tried to _____ the entire length of the hall by himself, but had to call for assistance halfway down.
    A. walk
    B. wake
    C. walking
    D. waking

47. Select the meaning of the underlined word in the sentence.
    The overt signs of the baby's illness were distressing to the parents.
    A. Easily observed
    B. Subtle
    C. Intestinal
    D. Feverish

48. The opposite of *contract* is _____.
    A. expand
    B. open
    C. mature
    D. obverse

49. Select the meaning of the underlined word in the sentence.
    <u>Exogenous</u> factors will affect the patient's well-being.
    A. Produced outside the body
    B. Produced within the body
    C. Produced by the kidneys
    D. Hereditary

50. Select the meaning of the underlined word in the sentence.
    <u>Endogenous</u> factors were responsible for his illness.
    A. Produced within the body
    B. Produced outside the body
    C. Polluting
    D. Hemocratic

51. Which word is not spelled correctly in the context of this sentence?
    The nurse went form room to room looking for the missing patient.
    A. patient
    B. form
    C. nurse
    D. missing

52. Which word is not spelled correctly in the context of the sentence?
    The physician thought it was unecessary to explain the procedure.
    A. physician
    B. unecessary
    C. explain
    D. procedure

53. Select the meaning of the underlined word in the sentence.
    The nurse observed that the skin around the sore was <u>inflamed</u>.
    A. Blanched
    B. Covered with a scab
    C. Cool to the touch
    D. Reddened

54. Select the word or phrase that makes this sentence grammatically correct.
    The child cried, "I want to do it _____!"
    A. mine
    B. me
    C. myself
    D. meself

55. Select the meaning of the underlined word in the sentence.
    His <u>paroxysmal</u> coughing was a sign of this illness.
    A. Occasional
    B. Convulsive
    C. Discreet
    D. Soft

56. Select the meaning of the underlined word in the sentence.
    The <u>potent</u> medication reduced the symptoms almost immediately.
    A. Correct
    B. Strong
    C. Liquid
    D. Tablet

57. Select the meaning of the underlined word in the sentence.
    The <u>precipitous</u> change was considered a good thing.
    A. Difficult
    B. Abrupt
    C. Gentle
    D. Unanticipated

58. Select the meaning of the underlined word in the sentence.
    The <u>rationale</u> for the therapy was to increase the patient's range of motion.
    A. Prescription
    B. Outcome
    C. Goal
    D. Reason

59. Select the meaning of the underlined word in the sentence.
    His <u>untoward</u> actions during the admission process created a problem for the nurse.
    A. Violent
    B. Casual
    C. Unseemly
    D. Capricious

60. Select the meaning of the underlined word in the sentence.
    The doctor's <u>verbal</u> prescription was implemented immediately.
    A. Narcotic
    B. Oral
    C. Written
    D. Current

61. What word is a synonym for *spit*?
    A. Expectorate
    B. Exfoliate
    C. Sputum
    D. Saliva

62. Which word is not spelled correctly in the context of the sentence?
    The ICU nurse-manger wanted all staff to sign the letter complaining about working hours at the unit.
    A. ICU
    B. sign
    C. manger
    D. complaining

63. Select the word or phrase that makes this sentence grammatically correct.
    The patient was _____ cold, so he asked the nurse for another blanket.
    A. not
    B. too
    C. to much
    D. so much

64. Which sentence is grammatically correct?
    A. She felt it was a breach of ethics to divulge the information.
    B. The pregnant woman was in danger of having a breach birth.
    C. The breech between the intestinal wall and urethra was life-threatening.
    D. The breech of confidentiality was reported to the head nurse.

65. Select the meaning of the underlined word in the sentence.
    The practical nurse is planning to administer a <u>transdermal</u> medication.
    A. Applied directly to the skin
    B. Injected just barely under the skin
    C. Injected in the tissue just below the skin layer
    D. Directly under the tongue

66. Select the meaning of the underlined word in the sentence.
    The bride decided to <u>expand</u> the number of people invited to the wedding.
    A. Decrease
    B. Increase
    C. Widen
    D. Reduce

67. Select the word or phrase that will make the sentence grammatically correct.
    The nurse completed the _____ incorrectly.
    A. from
    B. form
    C. pillow
    D. syringe

68. Select the meaning of the underlined word in the sentence.
    It is important that the bandage remain <u>intact</u>.
    A. Dry
    B. Whole
    C. Uncovered
    D. Secure

69. Select the correct meaning of the underlined word in the sentence.
    The office worker signed the <u>contract</u> for the new boss.
    A. Letter
    B. Receipt
    C. Agreement
    D. Card

70. Select the word or phrase in the sentence that is *not* used correctly.
    She has never tried to been in nursing school before.
    A. never tried
    B. tried to
    C. has never
    D. been in

71. Select the correct meaning of the underlined word in the sentence.
    The boys did not realize that their parents would be <u>accountable</u> for the boys' misbehavior.
    A. Unhappy
    B. Responsible
    C. Livid
    D. Keeping score

72. Which sentence is grammatically correct?
    A. Do you know when comes the bus?
    B. Do you know while bus comes?
    C. Do you know when the bus will come?
    D. Do you know how soon bus come?

73. Select the meaning of the underlined word in the sentence?
    The nurse told the patient, "You're so <u>obtuse</u>!"
    A. Overweight
    B. Ignorant
    C. Easy to read
    D. Uncaring

74. Select the meaning of the underlined word in the sentence.
    Being <u>bilingual</u> is an advantage for a nurse.
    A. Able to speak more than one language
    B. Able to use either hand with equal skill and ease
    C. Not squeamish when seeing blood
    D. Can remember everything that is read

75. Select the meaning of the underlined word in the sentence.
    The nurse is <u>accountable</u> for patient safety.
    A. Available
    B. Always aware
    C. Responsible
    D. Documenting

76. Why does a healthcare professional have a need for good grammar? (Select all that apply.)
    A. Charting must be accurate and concise.
    B. Patients and families are encouraged by fluency of the nurse.
    C. Good grammar helps the nurse better understand the instructions given.
    D. Good grammar is polite.
    E. Correct speaking is a sign of intelligence.
    F. Good grammar allows one to be able to correct the written errors of others.
    G. Good grammar allows one to be well liked by peers.

77. Select the word or phrase that makes this sentence grammatically correct.
    When will you be able to go the movies with _____?
    A. me
    B. I
    C. myself
    D. ourselves

78. Select the meaning of the underlined word in the sentence.
    The nurse noticed an <u>audible</u> gurgle when doing a physical examination on the patient.
    A. Observable
    B. Spasmodic
    C. Ominous
    D. Perceptible

79. Select the meaning of the underlined word in the sentence.
    The <u>parameters</u> of medical ethics require the nurse to report instances of suspected child abuse.
    A. Laws
    B. Limits
    C. Common sense
    D. Structure

80. Select the meaning of the underlined word in the sentence.
    To <u>alleviate</u> his pain, the nurse gave the patient a PRN medication.
    A. Pinpoint
    B. Relocate
    C. Eradicate
    D. Reduce

81. Select the meaning of the underlined word in the sentence.
    It is not wise to skimp on personal <u>hygiene</u>.
    A. Measures contributing to cleanliness and good health
    B. Financial resources available through the employment department
    C. Insurance
    D. Friendliness

82. Select the meaning of the underlined word in the sentence.
   The nurse noticed an <u>abrupt</u> change in the patient's level of pain.
   A. Slow
   B. Acute
   C. Subtle
   D. Sudden

83. Decomposition is the process of enzymes digesting food. Another name for this process is _____.
   A. degeneration
   B. dialysis
   C. lysis
   D. lymph

84. Select the word or phrase that will make the sentence grammatically correct.
   Because I want to go to the movies later, I am going _____ my homework now.
   A. doing
   B. to do
   C. be doing
   D. to doing

85. The patient fractured the lateral portion of the hip bone, which is known as the _____.
   A. ilium
   B. ileum
   C. icterus
   D. ileus

86. Tertiary health care might encompass which intervention?
   A. Early diagnosis
   B. Education about use of seat belts
   C. Community immunization programs
   D. Return to wellness

87. After a major heart attack, which assessment is most important?
   A. The patient's emotional adjustment to the heart attack
   B. The family and home problems
   C. Conditions that might impair cardiac functioning
   D. Factors that impair the client's well-being

88. Select the word or phrase in the sentence that is *not* used correctly.
   The data confirms that the patient is suffering from extreme anxiety, and a tranquilizing medication is immediately required.
   A. The data
   B. confirms
   C. is
   D. immediately

89. Which word can be defined as a truth, a rule, or a law?
   A. Prescription
   B. Tort
   C. Principle
   D. Malpractice

90. *Docile* is best defined as being _____.
   A. meek
   B. week
   C. firm
   D. tame

91. A person who is ravenous is _____.
   A. generous
   B. outspoken
   C. friendly
   D. hungry

92. Select the correct order of words to fit in the sentence structure.
   The nursing _____ put the Band-_____ on the wound to _____ the nurse.
   A. aid, aide, aide
   B. aide, aid, aid
   C. aid, aide, aid
   D. aide, aid, aide

93. Select the word or phrase that makes this sentence grammatically correct.
   He sat _____ Holly and Mary on the bus.
   A. though
   B. through
   C. among
   D. between

94. The word *spinster* is best defined as _____.
    A. a prim and proper person
    B. an unmarried woman
    C. a frequent traveler
    D. a greedy person

95. In the last election, 110,000 votes were cast. Candidate A received 60,000 votes, and 50,000 votes were divided between candidates B and C. Which statement indicates the outcome of this election?
    A. Candidate A has a plurality of 10,000 votes.
    B. Candidate B has fewer votes than candidate C.
    C. Candidate A has a majority of 10,000 votes.
    D. Candidate C has a minority of votes.

96. Based on Freud's theory, the "superego" _____.
    A. contains rigid rules
    B. is instinctive
    C. directs motor activity
    D. defines growth and development

97. Select the meaning of the underlined word in the sentence.
    Her <u>flushed</u> appearance was noted by the nurse during the examination.
    A. Pale
    B. Excited
    C. Ruddy
    D. Indifferent

98. Select the word or phrase that makes this sentence grammatically correct.
    The hospital is located at the top _____ the hill.
    A. in
    B. of
    C. on
    D. which

99. Select the word or phrase that will make the sentence grammatically correct.
    Within the _____ of the school, great emphasis is placed on participation in sports programs.
    A. confines
    B. milieu
    C. program
    D. brochure

100. Select the word or phrase that will make the sentence grammatically correct.
    The hunter has a _____ to *Field and Stream*.
    A. subscription
    B. prescription
    C. premonition
    D. consequence

101. Select the word or phrase that will make the sentence grammatically correct.
    _____ thought the movie was very good.
    A. Us
    B. We
    C. Wee
    D. Ourselves

102. Select the word or phrase that will make the sentence grammatically correct.
    The professor had a huge _____ of tests to grade.
    A. number
    B. amount
    C. aggregate
    D. stacks

103. Select the meaning of the underlined word in the sentence.
    The <u>proliferation</u> of text messaging among teens has alarmed parents.
    A. Increase
    B. Summarization
    C. Ambiance
    D. Rampant

104. What is the meaning of *laceration*?
    A. The best way to learn a new thing
    B. A deep, ragged tear
    C. Getting caught cheating
    D. Punishment

105. Select the correct meaning of the underlined word.
    The hot days of summer made the campers <u>lethargic</u>.
    A. Indolent
    B. Lazy
    C. Sleepy
    D. Energetic

Grammar and Vocabulary Answer Key

1. C		48. A	
2. B		49. A	
3. C		50. A	
4. A		51. B	
5. B		52. B	
6. B		53. D	
7. A		54. C	
8. B		55. B	
9. B		56. B	
10. B		57. B	
11. A		58. D	
12. C		59. C	
13. C		60. B	
14. B		61. A	
15. C		62. C	
16. B		63. B	
17. C		64. A	
18. A		65. A	
19. B		66. B	
20. D		67. B	
21. B		68. B	
22. B		69. C	
23. A		70. B	
24. A		71. B	
25. B		72. C	
26. B		73. B	
27. B		74. A	
28. A		75. C	
29. C		76. A, B, C	
30. B		77. A	
31. B		78. D	
32. A		79. B	
33. B		80. D	
34. B		81. A	
35. B		82. D	
36. A		83. C	
37. B		84. B	
38. C		85. A	
39. B		86. D	
40. B		87. D	
41. A		88. B	
42. C		89. C	
43. A		90. D	
44. B		91. D	
45. D		92. B	
46. A		93. D	
47. A		94. B	

95. C
96. A
97. C
98. B
99. B
100. A

101. B
102. A
103. A
104. B
105. C

ANATOMY AND PHYSIOLOGY, CHEMISTRY, AND BIOLOGY PRACTICE TEST

1. Within liver cells, glycogen can be decomposed to yield glucose. For this process to occur, which substances must also be present?
   A. Growth hormone and glucagon
   B. Insulin and corticosteroids
   C. Corticosteroids and epinephrine (adrenaline)
   D. Glucagon and epinephrine (adrenaline)

2. At which phase of meiosis does crossing over occur?
   A. Prophase I
   B. Prophase II
   C. Metaphase I
   D. Metaphase II

3. Which cellular process results in the formation of sugar from carbon dioxide?
   A. Krebs cycle
   B. Glycolysis
   C. Calvin cycle
   D. Cyclic phosphorylation

4. What is the name for the small, tail-like projection from the cellular membrane that is used for locomotion?
   A. Protein
   B. Basal body
   C. Flagella
   D. Actin

5. Which word refers to a region of the spinal cord?
   A. Lumbar
   B. Lumber
   C. Limber
   D. Limb

6. The phalanx is a(n)
   A. bone.
   B. joint.
   C. inflammation.
   D. opening.

7. The dermis is classified as a(n)
   A. cell.
   B. tissue.
   C. organ.
   D. system.

8. Upper motor neurons originate in which area of the body?
   A. Motor area of the cerebral hemispheres
   B. Anterior horns of the spinal cord
   C. Broca's area near the lateral fissure
   D. Within groups of skeletal muscles

9. Where are the pressoreceptors and chemoreceptors (specialized sensory nerves that assist with the regulation of circulation and respiration) located?
   A. Circle of Willis
   B. Cerebral arteries
   C. Abdominal aorta
   D. Carotid body

10. Where are the baroreceptors located?
    A. Lungs
    B. Aorta
    C. Heart
    D. Kidney

11. Which structure is an example of a long bone?
    A. Patella
    B. Cranium
    C. Vertebra
    D. Metatarsal

12. Which structure is divided into four lobes?
    A. Liver
    B. Mammary gland
    C. Lungs
    D. Cerebrum

13. Eye movement and papillary reflexes originate in which part of the central nervous system?
    A. Corpus callosum
    B. Hippocampus
    C. Midbrain
    D. Thalamus

14. Which vessel transports blood from the lung to the heart?
    A. Aorta
    B. Pulmonary artery
    C. Pulmonary vein
    D. Vena cava

15. What does the word *pulmonary* refer to?
    A. Lungs
    B. Heart
    C. Skin
    D. Liver

16. *Venous* refers to which body system?
    A. Circulation
    B. Respiration
    C. Digestion
    D. Autonomic

17. What is the primary sympathetic neurohormone?
    A. Acetylcholine
    B. Epinephrine
    C. Norepinephrine
    D. Dopamine

18. An improper balance between calcium and which substance can adversely affect the growth of healthy bone tissue?
    A. Chloride
    B. Sodium
    C. Phosphorus
    D. Magnesium

19. The function of the pulmonary veins is to carry
    A. unoxygenated blood to the lungs.
    B. oxygenated blood to the left atrium.
    C. unoxygenated blood to the pulmonary artery.
    D. oxygenated blood to the left ventricle.

20. What substance causes extreme dilation of arterioles and capillaries, stagnating blood flow within the tissues and leading to profound shock?
    A. Norepinephrine
    B. Ephedrine
    C. Histamine
    D. Nicotine

21. What is the expected pH of the stomach?
    A. 4.00 to 4.90
    B. 3.00 to 3.90
    C. 2.00 to 2.90
    D. 0.90 to 1.50

22. What mineral is responsible for muscle contraction?
    A. Chloride
    B. Sodium
    C. Calcium
    D. Magnesium

23. Bile is secreted into which organ?
    A. Small intestine
    B. Liver
    C. Large intestine
    D. Stomach

24. What is the function of glucocorticoids that are secreted from the adrenal cortex?
    A. To stimulate the secretion of HCL
    B. Carbohydrate, protein, and fat metabolism
    C. To regulate the "fight-or-flight" response
    D. Promotion of urinary functioning

25. What does parathyroid hormone regulate?
    A. Magnesium
    B. Calcium
    C. Calcitonin
    D. Glucocorticoids

26. What is the function of aldosterone?
    A. Converts proinsulin to insulin
    B. Conserves sodium in the body
    C. Protects against stress
    D. Affects heat production

27. What is the function of the baroreceptors?
    A. Increase urine excretion
    B. Increase rate of breathing
    C. Decrease heart rate
    D. Increase feelings of pain

28. Which nerve is responsible for regulating the amount of light entering the eye?
    A. Optic nerve
    B. Trochlear nerve
    C. Abducens nerve
    D. Oculomotor nerve

29. What component of the blood helps maintain glomerular oncotic pressure at a normal level of 33 mm Hg, which in turn keeps a large amount of water from escaping the capillary?
    A. Iron
    B. Fat
    C. Sodium
    D. Protein

30. Segments of a polypeptide chain can coil or fold as a result of hydrogen bonds, adding to a protein's structural conformation. What is this structure called?
    A. Primary structure
    B. Secondary structure
    C. Tertiary structure
    D. Quaternary structure

31. What is the concentration of 58.5 g of NaCl in 2 L of solution (atomic weights of each element are as follows: Na = 23 g/mol, Cl = 35.5 g/mol)?
    A. 0.5 mol NaCl
    B. 0.75 mol NaCl
    C. 1 mol NaCl
    D. 2 mol NaCl

32. What is the correct electron configuration for neon?
    A. 1s22s22p6
    B. 1s22s22p5
    C. 1s22s22p63s23
    D. 1s22s22p63s23p6

33. What is the ground state electron configuration for zinc?
    A. 1s22s22s63s23p64s23d10
    B. 1s22s22s63s23p64s23d9
    C. 1s22s22s63s23p64s23d8
    D. 1s22s22s63s23p64s2

34. What is a benefit of water's ability to make hydrogen bonds?
    A. Lack of cohesiveness
    B. Low surface tension
    C. Use as a nonpolar solvent
    D. High specific heat

35. What is the weakest of all the intermolecular forces?
    A. Dispersion
    B. Dipole interactions
    C. Hydrogen bonding
    D. Covalent bonding

36. What is the correct name of $MgSO_4$?
    A. Magnesium sulfate
    B. Manganese
    C. Manganese (II) silicate
    D. Magnesium sulfite

37. What is the correct formula for magnesium chloride?
    A. $MgCl_2$
    B. $MgCl$
    C. $Mg2Cl$
    D. Mg_2Cl_2

38. Phenolphthalein changes from colorless to pink in basic solutions. At what pH value would the solution remain colorless?
    A. 8.4
    B. 4.2
    C. 5.7
    D. 6.5

39. How could water be boiled at room temperature?
    A. Lower the pressure
    B. Increase the pressure
    C. Decrease the volume
    D. Raise the boiling point

40. Iodine and carbon dioxide undergo sublimation at room temperature and atmospheric pressure. What is this process?
    A. Changing from a gas to a solid
    B. Changing from a liquid to a gas
    C. Changing from a solid to a liquid
    D. Changing from a solid to a gas

41. A catalyst increases the rate of reaction by
    A. heating it up.
    B. increasing the entropy.
    C. increasing the enthalpy.
    D. lowering the activation energy.

42. Redox reactions are those that occur with a transfer of electrons. What would cause an increase in the oxidation number?
    A. Oxidation
    B. Solidification
    C. Reduction
    D. Neutralization

43. An experiment is performed to measure the temperature of boiling water at sea level. The actual boiling point is 100° C. The data taken during the experiment show values of 104.6° C, 104.5° C, and 104.5° C. What term best describes these data?
    A. Accurate
    B. Precise
    C. Variable
    D. Equivalent

44. Chemical reactions in living systems proceed along catabolic pathways, and there tends to be an increase in
    A. entropy.
    B. enthalpy.
    C. glucose.
    D. glycogen.

45. A diploid germ cell containing 72 chromosomes undergoes meiosis. How many chromosomes will be in each gamete?
    A. 18
    B. 36
    C. 72
    D. 144

46. What is the primary purpose of the flagella on the surface of cells?
    A. Movement of the cell
    B. Removal of cellular waste
    C. Replication of chromosomes
    D. Production of energy

47. What process is responsible for actively transporting small particles across the cell membrane?
    A. Hydrolysis
    B. Pinocytosis
    C. Diffusion
    D. Osmosis

48. What is the primary cause of water molecules moving into or out of the cell?
    A. Ion charge mismatch inside and outside the cell
    B. DNA strand mismatch along the cell membrane
    C. Water molecule pressure gradient along the cell membrane
    D. Enzymatic pressure gradient inside and outside the cell

49. Why is DNA important for metabolic activities of the cell?
    A. Initiates cellular mitosis
    B. Provides cell wall stability
    C. Increases glucose absorption
    D. Controls synthesis of enzymes

50. Which outcome measure would most likely indicate that a sample of water contains acid?
    A. pH
    B. Density
    C. Refraction
    D. Temperature

51. Which structure is the primary "control center" for cellular activities?
    A. Nucleus
    B. Lysosome
    C. Mitochondrion
    D. Endoplasmic reticulum

Science Answer Key

1. D		27. C	
2. A		28. D	
3. C		29. D	
4. C		30. B	
5. A		31. A	
6. A		32. A	
7. C		33. A	
8. A		34. D	
9. D		35. A	
10. B		36. A	
11. D		37. A	
12. A		38. A	
13. C		39. A	
14. C		40. D	
15. A		41. D	
16. A		42. A	
17. C		43. B	
18. C		44. A	
19. B		45. B	
20. C		46. A	
21. D		47. B	
22. C		48. C	
23. A		49. D	
24. B		50. A	
25. B		51. A	
26. B			

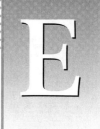

PHYSICS PRACTICE TEST

1. Which physical quantity is scalar in nature?
   A. 3:42 PM
   B. 23 m/sec; east
   C. 723 Nm; 216°
   D. 34 km/sec; sin (120°)

2. Determine the vertical component of a baseball's velocity if the ball is thrown at 28 m/sec at an angle of 37 degrees with the horizontal.
   A. 16.85 m/sec
   B. 22.36 m/sec
   C. 28 m/sec
   D. 21.2 m/sec

3. A hiker begins to move toward his chosen destination. He hikes 100 m east, 350 m north, 200 m west, 600 m south and 80 m east. What is his displacement along the y-axis as a result of this motion?
   A. 950 m; south
   B. 550 m; north
   C. 250 m; south
   D. 120 m; north

4. A bicycle trip of 680 meters takes 12.6 seconds. What is the average speed of the bicycle?
   A. 53.97 m/sec
   B. 8568 m-sec
   C. 0.054 km/min
   D. 8.57 m/sec

5. A go-cart has an initial speed of 23.4 m/sec. Fifteen seconds later the go-cart has a final speed of 46.8 m/sec. What is the magnitude of the go-cart's displacement?
   A. 702 m
   B. 526.5 m
   C. 362.7 m
   D. 877.5 m

6. You walk for 15 minutes at 3.8 m/sec and then decide to run for 12 minutes at 2.5 m/sec. What is your average speed?
   A. 3.22 m/sec
   B. 3.15 m/sec
   C. 13.5 m/sec
   D. 1.125 m/sec

7. A very strong young child tosses a stone into the air. His father times the stone's travel and finds that it takes the stone 2.8 seconds to return to the child's hand. How high did the stone rise?
   A. 27.44 m
   B. 13.72 m
   C. 9.60 m
   D. 31.36 m

8. A cannon is placed on the edge of a 300-meter-tall cliff. The barrel of the cannon is parallel to the ground below. If a cannonball leaves the barrel in a horizontal direction with a velocity of 115 m/sec, how far out from the base of the cliff will the cannonball land?
   A. 450.0 m
   B. 630.0 m
   C. 900.0 m
   D. 7,040.3 m

9. An object has a mass of 1,285 grams. Determine the weight of the object in newtons.
   A. 12,593 N
   B. 125.93 N
   C. 12.59 N
   D. 1,259.3 N

10. A car that weighs 15,000 N is initially moving at 60 km/hr when the brakes are applied. The car is brought to a stop in 30 m. Assuming the force applied by the brakes is constant, determine the magnitude of the braking force.
    A. 7,086.7 N
    B. 900,000 N
    C. 1,500,000 N
    D. 30,000 N

11. A hockey puck of mass 0.450 kg is sliding across the ice. The puck is initially moving at 28 m/sec. However, because of the frictional force between the puck and the ice, the motion of the puck is stopped in 15.8 seconds. Determine the magnitude of the frictional force.
    A. 1.65 N
    B. 7.81 N
    C. 0.80 N
    D. 5.49 N

12. A stone is tied to a 0.85-meter-long string and swung in a horizontal circle. If the stone makes one revolution every 0.50 seconds, what is the speed of the stone as it moves in this horizontal circle?
    A. 12.28 m/sec
    B. 6.28 m/sec
    C. 10,368 m/sec
    D. 5.24 m/sec

13. What is the kinetic energy of a 1,200-kg roadster moving at a rate of 88 km/hr?
    A. 9,292,800 J
    B. 105,600 J
    C. 358,519 J
    D. 52,800 J

14. An archer exerts a force of 15 N to pull back the bowstring 15 cm as she prepares to shoot an arrow. How much kinetic energy will be imparted to the arrow as a result of the work done?
    A. 225 J
    B. 112.5 J
    C. 2.25 J
    D. 1.125 J

15. A book of mass 0.95 kg is held 2.3 meters above the ground. Determine the gravitational potential energy of the book.
    A. 21.41 J
    B. 10.71 J
    C. 29.8 J
    D. 69.92 J

16. A 1,250-kg truck has a velocity of 28 m/sec to the east. What is the momentum of the truck?
    A. 17,500 kg-m/sec; east
    B. 35,000 kg-m/sec; west
    C. 35,000 kg-m/sec; east
    D. 17,500 kg-m/sec; west

17. A car of mass 1,350 kg experiences a force of 1500 N for 20 seconds. Determine the change in magnitude of the car's momentum.
    A. 15,000 N-sec
    B. 30,000 kg-m/sec
    C. 227,000 N-sec
    D. 101,250 kg-m/sec

18. A pendulum makes 12 vibrations every 60 seconds. What is the frequency of the pendulum?
    A. 5 Hz
    B. 0.083333 Hz
    C. 0.2 Hz
    D. 10 Hz

19. Three resistors are places in series. The resistors have values of 110 ohms, 45 ohms, and 60 ohms. Determine the value of the voltage needed to provide a current of 2 amp to this set of series resistors.
    A. 430 volts
    B. 220 volts
    C. 210 volts
    D. 107.5 volts

20. Electric fields are vector quantities because they are completely described by both magnitude and direction. According to scientific convention, the direction of an electric field is
    A. away from a positive charge.
    B. toward a positive charge.
    C. the direction a negative test charge would move when placed in an electric field.
    D. away from a negative charge.

21. When a concave mirror is used, where would an enlarged, virtual image be formed?
    A. At the focal point of the mirror
    B. Between the focal point and the mirror
    C. Behind the mirror
    D. At the center of curvature of the mirror

22. A certain ocean wave has a frequency of 0.05 Hz and a wavelength of 10 m. What is the wave's speed?
    A. 0.5 m/sec
    B. 200 m/sec
    C. 0.005 m/sec
    D. 100 m/sec

23. Sound is an example of _____.
    A. a longitudinal wave
    B. a transverse wave
    C. a standing wave
    D. a Doppler wave

24. An object has a weight of 6,000 N when resting on the surface of Earth. When located at a distance that is 3.2×10^7 m from the center of Earth, what is the new weight of the object? Remember that the radius of the Earth is 6.4×10^6 m and the mass of Earth is 6×10^{24} kg.
    A. 120 N
    B. 240 N
    C. 30,000 N
    D. 150,000 N

25. A spring is stretched 50 cm by a force of 1,000 N. What is the spring constant of this spring?
    A. 0.002 N/cm
    B. 0.05 N/cm
    C. 20 N/cm
    D. 500 N/cm

Physics Answer Key

1. A
2. D
3. C
4. A
5. B
6. A
7. C
8. C
9. C
10. A
11. C
12. C
13. C

14. C
15. A
16. C
17. B
18. C
19. A
20. A
21. C
22. A
23. A
24. B
25. C

INDEX

A

Abdominopelvic, definition of, 98
Abdominopelvic cavity, 90
Abrupt, definition of, 52
Absorption, definition of, 98
Abstain, definition of, 52
Abstract noun, definition of, 60
Acceleration
  centripetal, 110
  description of, 104
Access, definition of, 52
Accountable, definition of, 52
Acids, description of, 85
ACTH. *See* Adrenocorticotropic hormone
Actin, definition of, 98
Addition, 2-3
  of decimals, 8-10
  of fractions, 17-19
  of mixed numbers, 18
  with regrouping, 2
Adenine, deoxyribonucleic acid and, 77
Adenosine monophosphate, 94
Adenosine triphosphate
  cellular respiration and, 74
  definition of, 98
ADH. *See* Antidiuretic hormone
Adhere, definition of, 52
Adhesion, molecular, 72
Adjective
  description of, 60
  predicate, 62
Adrenocorticotropic hormone, 95
Adverb, description of, 61
Adverse, definition of, 52
Affect, definition of, 52
"Affect *vs.* effect," usage of, 66
Alleles, description of, 76

Alpha radiation, 82
Amino acid, definition of, 98
Amino acids, 73
  ribonucleic acid and production of, 77
"Among *vs.* between," usage of, 66
"Amount *vs.* number," usage of, 66-67
AMP. *See* Adenosine monophosphate
Amplitude
  definition of, 113b
  of wave, 114
Amylase, 96
Anaphase, cellular reproduction and, 75
Anatomy, 89-101
  general terminology of, 90
Annual, definition of, 52
Anterior direction, description of body and, 90
Antibody, definition of, 98
Antidiuretic hormone, 95
Antonym, context clues through, 47
Anus, role of, in digestion, 97f
Apply, definition of, 52
Arteries, 95
Arterioles, 95
Asexual reproduction, 75
Assumption, definition of, 48
Atom, description of, 81
Atomic mass, 81
  mole and, 83
Atomic number, 81
Atomic structure, 81
Atria, definition of, 98
Audible, definition of, 52
Audience, reading comprehension and, 47
Average speed, description of, 104
Axon, 94

B

"Bad *vs.* badly," usage of, 67
Bases, description of, 85
Beta radiation, 82
Bilateral, definition of, 52
Bile, definition of, 98
Binary fission, 75
Biology, 71-78
Blood, 95-96
Body, planes and directions of, 90
Bonding, chemical, 82-83
Bones
  description of, 91-93
  illustration of, 92f
Brain, 93
"Bring *vs.* take," usage of, 67

C

Calvin cycle, 75
"Can *vs.* may," usage of, 67
Capacity, conversion formulas for, 38
Carbohydrates, description of, 72
Carbon dioxide, respiration and, 96
Cardiac cycle, 95
Carpal bone, 91
Cartilage
  definition of, 98
  location of, 91
Case, pronoun, 63-64
Cast, definition of, 52
Catalyst, description of, 84
Cease, definition of, 52
Cell body, neuron and, 94
Cells
  description of, 73-74
  reproduction of, 75-76
Cellular membrane, description of, 74
Cellular respiration, 74

Page numbers followed by *b* indicate boxes; *f,* figures; *t,* tables.

Parameter, definition of, 54
Paroxysmal, definition of, 54
Parts of speech, 60
Patent, definition of, 54
Pedigree, definition of, 76
Pelvic girdle, 93
Percent, definition of, 32
Percent formula, 34-35
Percentages, 32-35
   decimal equivalents of, 37
   fractional equivalents of, 37
Periodic table, 80-81
Peripheral nervous system, 94
Personal pronoun, definition of, 60
pH
   definition of, 99
   description of, 85
Phagocytosis, definition of, 99
Phalanges, 93
Pharynx, role of, in digestion, 97f
Phospholipids
   in cellular membrane, 74
   description of, 72-73
Photosynthesis, description of,
   74-75
Phrase, description of, 62
Phylum, order of species and, 72
Physics, 103-118
Physiology, 89-101
   general terminology of, 90
Pituitary gland, 94
Place value
   in decimals, 8, 10
   definition of, 2, 28
   division of decimals and, 12
Plasma, 95
   definition of, 99
Platelets, 95
PNS. *See* Peripheral nervous system
Polarity
   chemical bonding and, 82
   of water, 72
Possessive case, description of, 63
Possessive pronoun
   contractions and, 65t
   definition of, 60
   description of, 63-64, 65b
Posterior direction, description of
   body and, 90
Potent, definition of, 54
Potential, definition of, 54
Potential energy, description of, 107
Precaution, definition of, 54
Precipitous, definition of, 55
Predicate, description of, 62
Predicate adjective, description
   of, 62

Predicate nominative, description
   of, 62
Predispose, definition of, 55
Preexisting, definition of, 55
Preposition
   description of, 61
   pronoun as object of, 64
   sentence ending with, 65
Primary, definition of, 55
Priority, definition of, 55
Product
   chemical equation and, 80
   definition of, 4
Profanity, elimination of, 66
Prognosis, definition of, 55
Projectile motion, description of,
   105-107
Prokaryotic cell, 73
Prometaphase, cellular
   reproduction and, 75
Pronoun
   case of, 63-64
   description of, 60
   reference of, 64
Proper noun, definition of, 60
Prophase, cellular reproduction
   and, 75
Proportion, 30-32
Protein
   deoxyribonucleic acid and
     production of, 77
   description of, 73
   synthesis of, deoxyribonucleic
     acid and, 77
Proton
   description of, 81
   electrical charge and, 116
Pulmonary circulation, definition
   of, 99
Punnett square, 76
Purpose, reading comprehension
   and, 47-48
Pyruvate, cellular respiration
   and, 74

Q
Quotient, definition of, 6, 12

R
Radiation, description of, 82
Radius bone, 91
Ratio, 30-32
Rationale, definition of, 55
Reactant, chemical equation and, 80
Reaction, types of, 80
Reading, 45-50
   critical, 48

"Reading between the lines," 48
Reciprocal, definition of, 23
Rectum, role of, in digestion, 97f
Recur, definition of, 55
Red blood cell, 95
Redox reaction, description of, 84
Reduction reaction, 84
Reflection, description of, 115
Refraction
   description of, 115
   lenses and, 115
Reproduction, cellular, 75-76
Reproductive system, 98
Resistance, Ohm's law and, 118
Resistor, electric circuits and, 118
Respiration, 96
   description of, 74
Respiratory system, 96
Restatement, context clues
   through, 47
Restrict, definition of, 55
Retain, definition of, 55
Ribonucleic acid
   description of, 73
   messenger, 77
Ribosome
   definition of, 99
   description of, 73
RNA. *See* Ribonucleic acid
Roman numerals, 38
Rotation, description of, 106
Run-on sentence, description of, 63

S
Sagittal, definition of, 99
Sagittal plane, description of body
   and, 90
Salivary gland, role of, in digestion,
   97f
Sarcomere, muscle function and, 93
Sarcoplasmic reticulum, definition
   of, 99
Scapula, 91
Sebaceous gland, 91
   definition of, 99
Second law of motion, 107
Sentence
   compound, 63
   description of, 62
   preposition at end of, 65
   run-on, 63
Sentence fragment, description
   of, 64
Serous membrane, 91
   definition of, 99
Sexist language, description of, 66
Sexual reproduction, 75-76